Gill Jacobs is a writer and sociologist with a background in research. She also teaches health education, relaxation and stress management. This is her first book.

CONTENTS

	Preface	vii
	Acknowledgments	ix
1	Introduction	1
2	Digestion	7
3	Understanding immunity	15
4	Jessica	19
5	What candida does	24
6	Allergies and food intolerance – paving the way	40
7	The candida war	46
8	Patterns of denial	57
9	ME in the media	67
10	Candida and ME: working in partnership	79
11	Stage by stage	84
12	Case histories – overload	88
13	Case histories – candida, tranquilliser addiction and antibiotics	94
14	Case histories – one symptom at a time	104
15	Case histories – turning points	111
16	Case histories – moving on	128
17	Case histories – men	135
18	Diagnosis and finding help	143
19	Rooting it out	147
20	Letting go of anger and fear, and taking control	168
	Information, support and advice	177
	Bibliography	185
	Index	187

But where danger is
Salvation grows as well.

Friedrich Hölderlin (1770–1843)

PREFACE

My initial motivation to write this book was a mixture of anger and curiosity. I wanted to find out whether a friend's harrowing experience with conventional medicine was an isolated one. Three years later, after talking to many other sufferers of candidiasis, I hope to demonstrate that it was not.

Stephanie, after a long and painful search for a diagnosis, eventually satisfied herself that she was suffering from a yeast condition known variously as candida or candidiasis. Her GP and the numerous consultants she had seen had not been able to help her, and this had caused whatever health problems she had to intensify. Eventually she recognised herself when she read an article on candida by the well-known naturopathic and osteopathic practitioner, Leon Chaitow.

At about this time I learnt that a relative had just discovered that candida was the cause of several years of extreme fatigue and debilitating health. Stephanie and I decided to find other candida sufferers and publicise their difficulties in order to increase awareness about the condition. Our first attempt – an advertisement in a local paper – produced only one reply. However, that interview convinced us that we were right to carry on, so we subsequently placed a request in the Action Against Allergy newsletter for sufferers to contact us. Within a week seventeen women replied, and over the next few months a few more, including one man. At this point my friend left the project to concentrate on other work, but she remained in the background with advice and support.

My previous experience as a sociologist had included a period interviewing school-leavers and their parents, using a method known as collaborative interviewing. Instead of questionnaires, certain areas were defined, but for the most part the respondents were allowed to bring up what was relevant in whatever way they chose. This became my approach to interviewing candida sufferers. It had the added advantage of giving me the chance to learn from others by letting them speak in their own way. It was only later that I realised how important that decision was. Many of the interviewees had suffered from not being able to talk about what was relevant to them, and the fact that interviewees were given the satisfaction of knowing that whatever they felt they needed to say was important to their story, proved of incalculable value.

Over the next three years I worked my way through the interviews, learning as I went along. In the beginning I was only interviewing women. Rapport seemed to come easily; although I didn't share their problems with candidiasis, there was an unspoken understanding between us as women about what it was like to be misunderstood or not listened to.

Later on when I interviewed male sufferers it was clear that medical failure to treat their candidiasis appropriately was equally devastating. A separate book needs to be written on the problems of candidiasis in children.

My biggest regret is that I have not been able to include all the material given to me. Each story had something to teach and I have done my best to include all the lessons they provided.

September 1989

I have taken advantage of this third impression to include new information in Chapter 19 on the treatment of candida. Feedback from candida sufferers suggests that many report feeling well while following the diet and taking anti-fungal supplements, but some find symptoms return when they cease treatment. New developments in candida control, particularly more effective probiotics and supplements to heal the gut should go some way towards tackling this problem.

ACKNOWLEDGMENTS

The initial impetus to write this book came from Stephanie Lehmann, whose own experience with candidiasis prompted my search for others. She was constantly in the background throughout this project, with encouragement, support and advice. Hetty Einzig provided a listening ear at various stages of writing. To them both I am particularly grateful. I am also greatly indebted to Mike Franklin for his early encouragement and practical advice.

The book could not have been written without the cooperation of all those I interviewed with candidiasis and ME who opened up their lives to my tape-recorder with such trust and generosity. I hope, however inadequately, I have been able to convey the extraordinary quality of what they gave me. It is impossible for me to name all those I interviewed or spoke to in the course of the research for this book, however indebted I am to them, but in particular I would like to thank four whose case studies do not appear in the book, but whose influence on the ideas within it was invaluable – Ann Pitman, Linda Howells, Sue Webster and Peter Wardley-Repen.

At a time when very little material on candidiasis was available in Britain, Dr William Crook, in the United States, sent me a copy of his book, *The Yeast Connection* (first published in 1983). His generosity led to a strengthening of my instinct to persevere against the conventional view. Of the many books I read, I would like to single out one in particular, although I do not refer to it in the text, *Intimate Partners: Patterns in Love and Marriage* by Maggie Scarf (Century Hutchinson, 1987), which taught me more than anything else how much could be gained from allowing others to do the talking.

I would like to thank the following people for giving me interviews about their approach to the treatment of candidiasis and ME: Dr Nadya Coates, Lily Cornford, Dr Stephen Davies, Dr Robert Erdmann, Dr Patrick Kingsley, Jo Hampton, Dr Harry Howell, Dr Jean Monro, and Dr John Stirling. Dr Kingsley and Dr Stirling were particularly helpful with comments on the scientific and medical data, and the ME chapters greatly benefited from being read and commented on by Dr Ellen Goudsmit and Doug Bullock.

I am of course aware that some of those who gave me their time and advice may not be in agreement with all my conclusions. I should therefore like to make it clear that I alone am responsible for them.

Lastly, I would like to thank the editor, David Symes, from whose professional expertise this book has greatly benefited. I would also like to thank my husband, Nick, for suggesting the quotation at the front of the book.

1 INTRODUCTION

It has been claimed that up to one-third of the total population of western industrialised nations suffer from illnesses in which yeast or *Candida albicans* is implicated.

Our bodies allow candida to wreak havoc when our immunity becomes weakened or when the balance of our intestinal ecology is distorted. This breach in our defences may start early in childhood, because of inherited deficiencies or a mother's inability to breastfeed. In recent years the huge increase in candidiasis has been encouraged by our overdependence on antibiotics and the birth control pill, the use of steroids and cortisone, and the decline in the quality of our diets. New evidence is emerging to link problems of immune function to electromagnetic interference. Our immunity is also affected by our emotions.

Unfortunately, candida sufferers are placed in a cruel dilemma – because doctors do not know about or do not recognise candidiasis, they easily attribute troublesome symptoms resistant to other diagnoses to stress. Stress is often a cofactor in the development of candidiasis, but in order to get better the organic basis of many of the symptoms has to be confronted too.

AN OPPORTUNISTIC INVADER

Candida albicans is a yeast mould which colonises our internal and external bodily surfaces (skin, mucosal surfaces and the digestive tract) not long after birth. It is important to realise that there are many different antigenic strains or types, all requiring a different response from our immune system when they get out of hand. Its favourite sites are the oesophagus and the small intestine. When kept in check it is commensal, i.e. it brings neither harm nor benefit to the host within which it lives. However candida is dimorphic – it can exist in two states. In the yeast form it can reproduce itself but is unable to move beyond the intestinal tract. If provided with ideal nutrients, though, and if allowed to multiply, it can transform itself into an invasive fungal form. It does this by producing mycelia, the intertwined threads commonly seen on fungi. Once changed in this way it uses the mycelia to penetrate the lining of the digestive tract, pushing out its root-like filaments to gain access to the bloodstream. The exact process by which candida becomes systemic needs further research.

Not only are other areas of the body open to colonization by the fungal form of candida, but the body must also cope with the resulting outflow of toxins from the candida cells. Excessive toxins further weaken the damaged mucosal linings in the gut, causing abnormal absorption of large protein molecules from the intestine into the bloodstream. The immune system, our body's way of defending against foreign invaders, becomes overworked; food allergies can result because of the immune system's reaction to undigested protein leaking through the gut. Clearly, the importance of early recognition is paramount.

Dr Nadya Coates, founder of the Springhill Cancer Centre, has developed interesting theories about the relationship of candidiasis to cancer, based on her own experience and her own and others' research. She believes that cancer will not develop unless there is candida overgrowth in the small intestines. The leaky gut produced by candida mycelia allow waste products excreted by bacteria to pass into the blood. Her view is that these substances are extremely carcinogenic, a view supported by the fact that cancerous tumours invariably include bacterial and fungal activity.

Candidiasis is seen by many clinical ecologists and holistic practitioners to be responsible for, or part of, many chronic and degenerative diseases, affecting almost all parts of the body, organs, tissues and cells. Symptoms include extreme fatigue and lethargy, headaches, cystitis and vaginitis, menstrual cramps and problems involving reproductive organs, gastrointestinal symptoms, skin problems, migraine, depression, muscle weakness and asthma.

Some doctors claim to have been successful in treating such diverse conditions as multiple sclerosis, endometriosis, autism, schizophrenia and arthritis when they recognised the role of candida and took steps to control it. Myalgic Encephalomyelitis (ME) and AIDS have been linked because of their similar viral involvement; but they also share problems of immunity, often with clear signs of candida infestation. As far back as the 1940s Dr Josef Issels wrote about the importance of balance in the ecology of the gastrointestinal tract, warning that an imbalance with candida growth was one of the causes of cancer.

On the other side are the sceptics who ridicule such comprehensive claims because of the lack of scientific evidence backed up by double blind trials and reliable diagnostic tests. The fact that the doctors so accused have been forced to break ranks and speak directly to the 'consumer' is used as evidence against them.

This book will not satisfy the call for 'controlled trials which have been approved for scientific merit and safety' (the Practice Standards Committee of the American Academy of Allergy and Immunology), but its aim is not to 'win' the argument with those means. No human being can be an acceptable control in such a medical trial for another human being, simply because candidiasis does not reproduce itself in the same way from one person to another. Moreover, double-blind controlled trials disallow clinical observation and patients' subjective feelings. 'Science' as the ultimate authority in medicine leaves out the unmeasurable facility of individual response and motivation.

One reason why many doctors still deny the role of candida is precisely because it does not fit their neater, more compact view of illness, which is organ specific and which does not demand an investigation into cause or the whole. This book asks an obvious question. Why is it that those who are trained to recognise and treat illness are also trained to close their eyes to new ideas, in spite of the evidence in terms of patient recovery? To be sure, in many instances we benefit from a cautious response to new ideas. But the history of 'scientific' medicine is stacked with other examples of imprudent haste, particularly in relation to drug therapy.

Sufferers of 'new' illnesses, such as candidiasis, are usually forced to rely on magazines, self-help books and the media for their diagnosis and treatment. We must assume that doctors have the same exposure to these sources of information as the rest of us; what is clear is that these sources are considered by the medical profession to be unscientific and uninformed. Medical school lecture notes, what little there are of them when it comes to microbiology, remain selectively sacred in this particular instance.

But the 'war' is not so clearcut, and teasing out what is acceptable and scientifically proven opens up the possibility of convergence. Conventional doctors do not deny that *Candida albicans*, and other forms of fungi, can do damage in the body, but they only see that damage in two situations. Firstly when it surfaces, as with vaginal and oral thrush and skin infections (the textbooks are liberally provided with extreme illustrations of candida in its most virulent form). And secondly when it has become systemic, usually as a result of medical intervention for other conditions. There is a sizeable literature on systemic candidiasis and its life-threatening potential in people who are, for example, receiving powerful drugs for the treatment of leukaemia and other cancers. In these cases the immune system has been suppressed by the drugs that are given to fight the cancer, and candida is free to spread.

Candidiasis, until recently, was difficult to test for. The textbooks reveal that doctors have the tricky dilemma of knowing that it is likely in certain situations, but having to decide whether to hold back from applying antifungal chemotherapy without scientific evidence of its need, because the toxicity of the drugs is only worth risking on those who definitely require them. The reality of the situation is that doctors only know who definitely requires treatment after they are dead, although some clinical ecologists and candida practitioners now use tests which claim to identify the presence of systemic candidiasis. These tests have been slow to be recognised within scientific medicine. One is bound to speculate as to what the major cause of death might have been – cancer *per se*, organs pickled by yeast, or liver and kidney damage from the drugs given for candida, after the drugs given for cancer.

At the heart of this dilemma is the obvious question – if something is present in a chronic way, brought about by extreme iatrogenic provocation (i.e. caused by the treatment of other diseases), is it not possible for it also to be present in a less dramatic way, developing over many years and with many causes?

In other illnesses we do not wait for external visible signs of disease. We spend much effort and scientific energy devising means to assess what is going on internally. We take it for granted that tumours can grow unseen and unfelt. Why then do we see a role for candida only when it shows itself externally and is directly testable, or when it has become chronic throughout an already decaying body? What about the stages in between?

It is not hard for women, who form the majority of sufferers from candidiasis, to find other examples to parallel conventional scepticism and convenient prejudice. We have been in the front line as sufferers of unclassifiable symptoms. Thus we used to be told by doctors that our problems with premenstrual tension were psychological: now premenstrual tension, and its organic basis in hormonal irregularity, is accepted enough to be used in a court of law as a defence for anti-social behaviour. To take one more step and consider the possibility that such irregularity could be caused by an underlying problem with candida, because of its effect on hormone regulation, is still a long way off.

Those who do acknowledge the role of candida are not saying that all the symptoms associated with it are caused by candida. Indeed most practitioners who treat candida are careful to point out that it usually accompanies other pre-existing problems. Alternatively, symptoms attributed to candidiasis could be caused by other factors, such as intestinal parasites.

Thus far into the argument you may still be thinking that this is another passing fad, another single solution for a host of totally unrelated illnesses. Your response to the rest of the book will depend initially on how you see illness and disease. Much has been written recently opposing holistic to 'scientific' medicine. Candida can only be understood in the context of an overall view of health which takes account of the connections between the mind and the body, and the environment which affects them both. It is not 'holistic' to view dis-ease in simplistic terms. But candida becomes more acceptable as an explanation if it is seen to partner other bio-chemical processes which need adjusting, all uniquely combined in each individual.

With the help of numerous case studies, I want to dispel the sense of hopelessness and despair that many sufferers of candidiasis and ME experience. Candidiasis usually responds to treatment over time, as long as underlying deficiencies and problems are tackled as well. The problem for many has been the lack of recognition, piecemeal treatment, disillusion when trying to rely solely on diet, and damage done by over-enthusiastic use of antifungal drugs.

Reading the case material it is clear that this story does not have neat divisions between the 'goodies' outside conventional medicine and the 'baddies' within. Some of the interviewees had candidiasis diagnosed as patients of NHS allergy clinics; others pay tribute to their GPs, who may not have known about candidiasis but who nevertheless provided support and encouragement when it was desperately needed. Although I tried to place critical comments about doctors and therapists in a balanced perspective, I noted that those with critical comments were also those most ready to acknowledge positive interventions and help where appropriate.

It is no exaggeration to say that thousands of people in Britain today are ill without knowing the cause; others have been wrongly diagnosed and fail to recover. Because they do not come to the notice of doctors who may provoke their candida into systemic virulence in situations which are recognised, they fall through the net of authenticity. Because the host of possible symptoms seems to gather together most of the problems which modern medicine has failed to help, the theory is then dismissable because it is 'unlikely'. Rather than dismiss candida straightaway, it would seem worthwhile to try and find out more, at least to make an informed choice before its diagnostic value is denied to potential sufferers.

2
DIGESTION

Candida albicans is just one of the many microorganisms – the flora – which live on and in us. In simple terms these microorganisms can be divided into viruses, bacteria, fungi and minute single-celled organisms called protozoans, of which the bacteria and fungi predominate in the gut. Our indigenous gut flora consists of about 3–4 lb of bacteria, with 300–500 species, for the most part concentrated in the large intestine; it has been estimated that these microorganisms form approximately half of all our stools.

The bacteria and other organisms in our gut perform many important metabolic functions, and are thus essential to our healthy functioning. Our intestinal ecology depends on a delicate balance between all these various microorganisms; if some species start to proliferate at the expense of others, it can have serious implications for our health.

One of the most beneficial, yet also the most vulnerable, of the bacteria are the bifidobacteria. They help to maintain an acidic pH in the large intestine, thus deterring any imbalance occurring from an overgrowth of invading pathogens (disease-causing organisms), including the fungal form of *Candida albicans*.

Lactobacillus acidophilus, as its name implies, thrives in an acidic environment, as produced by the bifidobacteria. If acidophilus is present in sufficient numbers in the large intestine it will prevent any overgrowth by yeasts. Milk is turned into yogurt partly through the action of acidophilus, making yogurt a beneficial food in the battle against unfriendly microorganisms in the gut.

Lactobacillus acidophilus has the ability to break down milk sugar (lactose), something that the digestive systems of many adults cannot do. Breastfeeding a baby encourages the growth of acidophilus in the baby's gut, supplementing the protection that breastmilk automatically confers. Some of the candida sufferers that I interviewed were fed sugared water from birth, which could well have been the start of their problems with candida.

Our intestinal flora also protects the condition of the mucosal wall of the gut, across which nutrients pass into the bloodstream. This is very important if we are to prevent candida becoming systemic, i.e. prevalent throughout the body. Moreover, if candida overgrowth does occur there is a possibility that the gut wall will become impacted with hardened material consisting of dead organisms – yeasts, bacteria, etc. – mucus and faecal material, thus limiting the passage of nutrients into the bloodstream.

In *Tissue Cleansing through Bowel Management* Bernard Jensen summarises the beneficial effects of friendly bacteria in the following way.

> When we properly care for the bowel, we are automatically providing a welcome home for those favourable life-giving bacteria that are essential to good health. Among other things they provide very valuable nutritional metabolites for the body to use in rebuilding and maintaining health. Examples are portions of the vitamin B complex, enzymes and essential amino acids, the increased and more efficient absorption of calcium, phosphorus and magnesium. They are responsible for the synthesis of certain vitamins. They maintain an antibacillus coli environment. They contribute to health in many ways we are not scientifically aware of yet.

HOW WE DIGEST FOOD

Most people with candida at some stage experience problems with digestion. In the process of unravelling the cause of candidiasis it is important to look at how we digest food to provide nourishment for the rest of the body. Knowing what can go wrong is essential if we are to take steps to correct any imbalance.

Before we look at the mechanics of digestion, though, it is of value to understand the basic processes underlying it. The food we eat consists for the most part of large complex molecules; the process of digestion is to break down these large molecules into small molecules which can pass across the gut wall into the bloodstream, in which they are then transported to the organs where they are needed to fuel our body chemistry or metabolism. The breakdown of the large molecules is achieved by enzymes, different enzymes breaking down different groups of foods – some enzymes break down proteins, some break down specific carbohydrates, some break down larger groups of carbohydrates, some break down fats.

Enzymes operate best under optimum conditions; for example, all our digestive enzymes function best at body temperature. However, our different digestive enzymes also operate best at various levels of acidity or alkalinity; for example, under ordinary circumstances this means that enzymes from the stomach, which is acidic, will not work once they reach the small intestine, which is alkaline. The levels of acidity are measured on the pH scale, whereby increasing acidity is measured from 7 to 1, increasing alkalinity from 7 to 14, and 7 indicates neutrality.

Various digestive juices ensure that different sections of the alimentary tract are at the correct pH for the different digestive enzymes to function, and beneficial microorganisms, particularly in the intestines, can reinforce this control. However, if harmful microorganisms get a chance to proliferate they can upset this important balance.

The process of digestion commences in the mouth. Here the chewing action breaks down the lumps of food into small particles on which subsequent digestive juices can act more efficiently. The food particles are also mixed with fluid, which lubricates the passage of the food down the throat into the stomach. The fluid provides a slightly acidic environment, in which a salivary enzyme can work to best advantage, starting the breakdown of some starchy foods.

The food then reaches the stomach. The sight of food, the action of chewing and then the arrival of the food in the stomach will all have stimulated the production of the digestive juices. These juices produce a very acidic environment, which quickly inactivates the salivary enzyme but which provides optimum conditions for the gastric enzymes (which digest proteins). The high acidity also serves to kill off any putrefying bacteria which might have been ingested with the food.

However, if there is too little acid and pepsin (the gastric enzyme) produced, fermentation can occur if yeasts or other microorganisms get a foothold. Dr Erdmann estimates that as many as nine out of ten stomach upsets are wrongly attributed to too much acid, the real cause being the reverse – too little acid, leading to fermentation of the stomach contents. The common practice of taking antacids – compounds that reduce the acidity in the stomach – for indigestion is therefore not necessarily the correct course of action in all cases, and can even aggravate the problem, as well as interfere with the absorption of essential nutrients such as calcium, magnesium, iron and phosphorus.

In this respect, our own biological individuality should not be under-emphasised. Stomachs differ widely in size and shape, and in the composition of their digestive juices. It has been found that there can be as much as a thousandfold variation in the pepsin (the protein-digesting enzyme) content of the gastric juices, and our ability to function with high or low levels of pepsin also appears to vary.

In the stomach the mass of food very quickly becomes a liquid and is churned around before being passed on into the upper reaches of the small intestine, this region being called the duodenum. And it is into the duodenum that the majority of the digestive enzymes are secreted. The pancreas secretes enzymes that continue the digestion of proteins begun in the stomach, as well as producing two other enzymes that break down fats and some carbohydrates. The duodenal wall produces a wide variety of digestive enzymes that break down many different carbohydrates, variously partially digested protein units, some fats and various other nutrients. And from the liver, via the gallbladder, comes bile that helps in the digestion of fats. All these juices are alkaline, and the enzymes they contain function best at a neutral or slightly alkaline pH.

In general, very few nutrients are absorbed from the stomach, principally because the process of digestion has not proceeded far enough at that stage. As the mixture of food and digestive juices passes along the small intestine the nutrients are broken down into smaller and smaller units and are absorbed into the bloodstream. Then, from the small intestine, the food mass passes into the large intestine, whose principal task is to absorb water from the waste products of digestion. However the large intestine also contains large quantities of microorganisms, as already explained, and they assist in the final stages of digestion. For example, there are bacteria which assist in the synthesis of chemical compounds such as vitamins and the essential colonic fatty acid, butyric acid.

We have already seen how, if the acidity and activity of the gastric juices in the stomach are too low, putrefactive bacteria and yeasts, ingested with our food, can start to proliferate. When such a mass of poorly digested fermenting food passes on into the small intestine, the whole system can become overwhelmed and fail to secrete enough digestive enzymes to prevent further fermentation and putrefaction. The result can be excess mucus production, diarrhoea and ultimately the development of allergies. Furthermore, the process of fermentation and putrefaction can produce various alcohols which are absorbed into the bloodstream. These alcohols can then interfere with blood-sugar levels, with the result that you feel fatigued and lacking in energy.

If candida overgrowth goes too far there is the chance of it changing to its mycelial, fungal form and penetrating the intestinal wall. If this occurs the so-called 'colander effect' can allow undigested protein to enter the bloodstream. This is an abnormal state of affairs, as the body cannot tolerate or process protein in this form, and sometimes responds with an allergic reaction.

A PROCESS OF ELIMINATION

The way we handle waste is becoming a topic that has to be taken seriously. Governments are belatedly being forced to recognise that we cannot have the benefits of an industrial and nuclear society without at the same time being responsible for the destruction and degeneration that their emissions and waste products cause. A few years ago the ozone layer was not part of the general vocabulary – now most school children are aware that their futures are threatened by our irresponsible attitude to survival.

When it comes to our own organs of waste disposal we have been equally slow to realise their importance. This is partly because those that have recognised the basis of much disease in poor bowel management have been thought of as cranks. Sir Arbuthnot Lane (1856–1943) earned the reputation of being one of the best surgeons of his time. But his belief in the centrality of the colon and its ability to cause many illnesses throughout the body is singled out as an example of 'prejudice and irrational practice' in the medical profession by Dr Glin Bennet in his book *The Wound and the Doctor*. Sir Arbuthnot Lane argued that slow elimination of waste created kinks in the intestinal tract, which then harboured toxic debris and caused inflammation, ulceration and cancer. The toxins could spread to other areas of the body by absorption, leading to, among other problems, degeneration of the heart, arteries, kidneys and muscle, and problems of blood pressure and mental illness.

> This is a formidable list of complaints to ascribe to a single cause, and worthy of any quack dominated by an idea offering an explanation for so many human ills. Lane, however, saw himself as entirely rational: and of course he was, except for his initial false premise concerning the noxious effects of the imaginary condition – alimentary toxaemia. *The Wound and the Doctor* Glin Bennet

If this is typical of a wider avoidance of the colon's importance, because it is claiming too much, it is easy to see how many medical practitioners also reject the possibility of candida being responsible for an equal amount of disease in the body.

We might be justified in thinking that Lane's theories were an elaborate ruse to allow him to practise what he was most skilled at – surgery, and in particular the removal of the colon. For example, at a meeting on alimentary toxaemia before the Royal Society of Medicine in 1911, Lane reported a case where a surgeon had proposed an operation for the removal of a tumour from the frontal lobe of the brain. The need for this was avoided by the excision of the colon. However, having proved to himself that other problems went away when the colon was removed, by observing what happened to patients, he sensibly reasoned that such interventions could be bypassed if patients could be persuaded to change their diets. He campaigned against white bread, and set up the New Health Society, but it was to be many years before anyone took his views seriously and, as we can see above, there is still a difficulty about linking different parts of the body together in a coherent and rational view of the cause of toxicity and degeneration.

Once vegetable matter has been digested there is little left apart from the fibrous material, which passes through the gut unaffected by the digestive process. In contrast, meat is not digested quite so efficiently, and residues can remain in the intestines where they can provide a focus for putrefactive bacteria; undesirable byproducts can result and then can be asborbed by the body. Limitation of this problem can be achieved if there is a rapid bowel transit time, i.e. if the residues of digestion pass through the large intestine fairly swiftly.

If the processing of waste matter in our large intestine needs to be fast, it is essential that our diets include enough fibre to gather up toxic waste. Fibre, which we cannot absorb, can gather up organisms that are potentially harmful, before they become established in the bowel wall. Fibre is the undigestible part of what we eat. It is important because it affects the transit time of the food in the digestive tract. A normal and beneficial transit time would be from 24 to 48 hours, but if the fibre content of food is low this time can be greatly increased. One result of a lengthy transit time is that water loss from faeces through the intestinal wall is increased, leading to hard stools and constipation. Another result could be the creation of small pockets in the intestinal wall where deposits of decaying material and bacteria are left behind; the condition called diverticulitis can then erupt, whereby the pouches become inflamed with the accumulation of toxins. Yeasts can also flourish on such dead and decaying matter.

Fibre is best provided by fruit and vegetables, and whole grains like brown rice, wholewheat and oats. However, fibre from wheat is not beneficial to candida sufferers because it contains particles of bran in which there is gluten, fungus and environmental toxins. Dr Coates (see page 149) is particularly cautious about gluten, maintaining that a porous gut allows gluten into the bloodstream and thence to organs such as the liver, pancreas and gallbladder, causing disturbed function (this is because gluten is sticky, adhering to surfaces). In addition to these reasons, adding wheatbran to food is not a sensible way of ensuring more fibre because it causes a scraping action on the lining of the gastrointestinal tract, leading to irritation and diarrhoea. It also raises sugar levels and lowers absorption of minerals such as magnesium and zinc. Oatbran is a better alternative.

Meat, fat and sugar between them only contributed 15 per cent of the total amount of calories in the diet a hundred years ago; now, that percentage has risen to nearly 60 per cent. Correspondingly, what has declined is the amount of fruit and vegetables and cereals, all of which contribute fibre to the diet. It is not surprising, then, that problems with the colon should be so widespread. What is surprising is that so little attention is paid to the consequences of poor digestion and bowel management as they relate to disease throughout the body.

DIGGING DEEPER FOR THE BROADER VIEW

Mapping out the territory in which candida lives and grows makes it easier to understand the wider complexities of life in the gut. By looking behind the growth of candida and following the process of digestion, it is easier to understand what happens later. Behind each interaction is another one, and behind that is something else, and they are all interdependent and all capable of affecting the chain of events.

Some of the symptoms attributed to candida are more accurately derived from disruption of the digestive process. It is convenient for the moment to talk of the symptoms as caused by candidiasis, but it may be more useful in the long term to take a broader view which encompasses all the disturbances caused by digestive processes which have gone wrong.

3 UNDERSTANDING IMMUNITY

So far we have concentrated on one aspect of candida growth – digestion and the acid/alkaline balance in the gut, only touching on some of the others. But no understanding of candida overgrowth is complete without a working knowledge of how the immune system functions. The problem for a person with candidiasis is with the immune defence system just as much as with yeast overgrowth itself.

We are surrounded by potential invaders – viruses, bacteria, fungi, other parasites, chemicals, dust, pollens, improperly degraded food – all trying to get past our defences, and often succeeding because of weakened resistance. Grouped together, these invaders can all be called antigens; if they get into the body they should provoke an immune response that will either dispose of them or limit their damage.

However, we are all different, we all possess individual variability of immune function; no two people can have the same disease in the same way, and this applies equally to candidiasis. The medical model is unable to account for the fact that some groups of people are more susceptible than others to illness of all kinds. Thus the antibiotic mentality changed medical thinking to look for the magic bullet to cure every disease, rather than consider the total context in which the illness is manifest.

Michael Weiner in his book *Maximum Immunity* suggests that the most powerful weapons to strengthen our resistance to illness are the mind, the food we eat, the exercise we follow and the rest we take. Unfortunately, he continues, modern man is overweight and malnourished, overstressed and unfit. The effects of the environment should also be added to this list – much recent research is pointing to the harmful effects on our immune systems of electromagnetic fields and chemical pollutants.

Every aspect of disease is affected by the healthy functioning of our immune system, because the immune system controls the body's total response to illness, from the early stages to the final throes of battle. Learning how to boost immunity is essential in the fight for recovery from illness, and in the maintenance of healthy balance.

A few of the people contributing to this book were fascinated to notice that one of the first signs of their recovery was their increased reaction to an infection, such as a cold. They learnt to greet a fever with joy and optimism as a sign that at last their internal defences were starting to mobilise. When their immune systems were weaker they did not respond to infection with fever in the normal way. Dr Charles Sheppard in his book *Living with ME* admits that in his own experience with ME he never succumbs to an infection with a raised temperature, but just feels cold and shivery. Seeing this as a 'strange aspect' of temperature control, he misses the connection with poor immune functioning. Dr Josef Issels reported this relationship as far back as 1948.

HOW THE IMMUNE SYSTEM WORKS

The immune system is made up of specialised organs and cells. The primary organs are the thymus and the bone marrow; the secondary organs include the lymph nodes, spleen, tonsils, appendix, Peyer's patches in the small intestine, and small specialised lymph nodules in the membranes of the intestines. Lymph areas become swollen in the presence of infection; thus when the tonsils become swollen it is a sign that something is wrong, not that they should be removed and prevented from further work.

The white blood cells are the active constituents of the immune system, and divide into three – B cells, T cells and macrophages. Together the T and B cells are called lymphocytes. B cells, coming from the bone marrow, produce antibodies (or immunoglobulins) that are released into the body fluids to fight antigens or foreign invaders. This is called our humoral immunity. We are protected from diseases that we have had in the past, or for which we have had immunisations, by 'memory' cells that allow a fast antibody response to a familiar antigen.

T cells are produced in the thymus gland (which is to be

found just below your breast bone) and they are responsible for cell mediated immunity; that is, they do not produce antibodies themselves, but they can remove antigens and influence other white blood cells to enter the fray. The following is a graphic description of how this part of the immune system is triggered into action.

> Imagine the T-cell response as an army, divided by the thymus into regiments of cavalry, infantry and heavy artillery. Looking at each 'regiment' at a time, the cavalry are those T-cells called lymphocytes. As the army's vanguard, they circulate rapidly around the body, reconnoitring the territory, always looking out for foreign invaders. They are extremely mobile, taking advantage of the interrelationship of every part of the body with every other part. A T-cell can easily travel from a brain neuron to a cell in your little toe. It uses the main arteries and veins of the circulatory system before slipping into smaller blood vessels and finally down into the capillaries. From here it will cross into the space between blood and the cell wall. Once it makes contact with the wall, the T-cell will examine it for signs of damage or infection. If the coast is clear it will leave the cell to travel elsewhere.
>
> When lymphocytes do locate an invader they call up other regiments of their army. The first to arrive is the infantry, a group of amino-derived hormones called lymphokines. These are thought to be the body's own natural drugs and include the well-known chemical interferon. They battle with micro-organisms and toxic chemicals, breaking them down into harmless parts which the body can dispose of. If the invader is larger, the heavy artillery is brought into action – the macrophages. Literally translated, macrophage means 'big eater' and this is exactly how it works, engulfing the invader before secreting an enzyme to destroy it.
>
> R. Erdmann and M. Jones, *The Amino Revolution*

In addition to the three T-cell units there are also T-helper and T-suppressor cells. Helpers are called up when needed, and these alert the B-cells to produce antibodies. Suppressors are essential to regulate the amount of antibody production; without the T-suppressor cells the other immune cells engaged in aggressive action against antigens might carry on fighting when their job is finished. Thus T-suppressor cells prevent the war being an own-goal, saving the body's own cells from destruction.

The normal ratio of helper to suppressor cells is 1.8:1, and any variations around this average give an indication of improper functioning of the immune system. AIDS patients usually have a ratio of 1:1 or less, indicating that the suppressor cells have increased beyond a safe level. The effect of this is to detune the immune system so that it is not alert enough to defend the body. The opposite situation would be autoimmune diseases, in which the T-suppressor cells are too few.

Underpinning all these processes are the building blocks of the body's protein structure, and the raw materials for immune functioning – amino acids. The immune cells and their products are made from amino acids, relying at the same time on vitamins such as vitamin C and the B complex and trace elements. And so we come full circle, back to the nourishment we give ourselves and how we process it.

4
JESSICA

Jessica's was the first interview. In the light of the other interviews, her recovery was surprisingly uncomplicated once she had found out about candidiasis. Because of this she is not representative of many of the other interviews in the book. In her case, candidiasis did not seem to be part of a childhood history of weakened immunity. Nystatin is only effective against two of the many strains of candida and she clearly had one of them. Her problems with diagnosis were not isolated, however. When she first got ill in 1980 there were very few doctors in Britain who had heard of candidiasis.

My stomach used to bloat. If I was wearing anything around my waist at all I'd get a horrible headache up the side of my head and I'd get incredibly tired. I dealt with it by wearing baggy dresses. Even though I'm quite slim, I'd look four or five months' pregnant.

It started just after I got married in the summer of 1980. I'd done my finals and lived a very unhealthy few months. I don't know whether it was connected with that but I was eating rubbish and smoking very heavily. I don't think I was eating much sugar, just no vegetables and greens, and drinking a lot of coffee. It was a very stressful time for me, and that's why I was eating badly. I lost a lot of weight and was very run down.

I always do much worse at exams than I should do. I was working hard but I knew all along it was to no effect, although in the end I got a 2.2. Also I wasn't living with my fiancé. I'd lived with him for two years before that and he had gone off to do his MSc, so he was ignoring me quite a lot.

My parents are both psychoanalysts, so it was natural for me to think it was psychological. I'd been analysed, and I thought it was stress or something like that. But only my intellectual side thought that. My other side didn't think it was really because it didn't seem to relate at all. So I went back to see my analyst for one day a week, entirely because of it. Because it was so unpleasant to have, I thought I should try and control it.

She was very reasonable about it and undogmatic. She tried to help me, but she thought it might be physical, and she encouraged me quite a lot to go to doctors, which is what I did. At first I went to my GP who took it quite seriously. I don't know why. I must have impressed her. She sent me off to a consultant, a general physician. He thought it might be hyperthyroidism because I had slightly strange anaemia, large blood cells. Anyway he decided that it wasn't that, and that it was irritable bowel. I wasn't convinced by this at all because it didn't sound like my symptoms.

They gave me this medicine that makes you go to the lavatory a lot, and that was not my problem at all. It was absolutely unrelated. And so I gave up with that. Then I left it for a while, and then after another year I got completely fed up with feeling bloated. I wasn't very well at all. Now that I feel so much better I realise. I had two days of bloating the other week and I just felt terrible. I felt very tired and slightly headachey. I used to be exhausted all the time. I just wanted to lie down. It wasn't just feeling sleepy, it was total exhaustion.

I was usually a little better in the morning and then after I'd had breakfast (toast) it was always a downhill thing. So I went back to my GP and said I can't bear it, it must be something. I was convinced it wasn't just psychological. So she sent me off to another consultant at another hospital who was much nicer but he still couldn't diagnose it. He said to try malabsorption, because the other problem was I was anaemic. I'd had my first child by then. He was born in 1982.

After the birth I felt dreadfully run down. I didn't eat enough after and during the pregnancy. I should have forced myself to eat much more. I thought it didn't matter because one of the books on pregnancy says the baby gets everything. I was so anaemic and so tired that I didn't have any appetite. It wasn't a straightforward pregnancy, though I can't imagine how that is connected.

The doctors were very worried about the baby because he had eight scans. They thought he might be underweight because I only put on 7 pounds. I'm sure that wasn't good for him, all those scans, and after the birth he was badly jaundiced. He had to go under a light for quite a long time. He was too weak to suck but I managed to pump my milk and eventually he was able to feed. He was so weak when he was born. It was a horrible birth. They yanked him out and I wouldn't have minded if he had died, frankly. Horrible.

My anaemia had got worse during the pregnancy and I hadn't responded to the iron. My second consultant decided that it wasn't malabsorption but irritable bowel. When he described it, it just sounded much more like what I thought I had because he described my symptoms back to me. So I said, well, maybe it is. And that was that. I basically decided I had to live with it. They kept testing me for different sorts of blood problems, trying to connect the blood with the stomach problem, because there are diseases that connect. But when they decided that I had irritable bowel I think they basically said there is nothing we can do for it. They gave me these fibo-gel things, which I'd had before. I don't think they did anything. I think he just said I'm sorry, that's it, sort of thing, nobody knows why you get it, and gave me a little talk, what it's to do with, and that it might be to do with stress. My son was seven months by this time. Then I went back a couple of times when it became clear that it wasn't whatever else he was trying to prove it was. I think I then just decided to ignore it again, for another year or two.

I tried going to a homoeopath but that was no good at all. So then I gave up again. My mother-in-law kept saying that I must go and see this allergist, and on top of that I kept refusing because I didn't really believe in that sort of thing. Then I saw this programme on television about irritable bowel, a lot of it being to do with allergies. It was also in the press. I got quite excited by that, and went off to my GP and said that I wanted to see the doctor on the programme, Dr Jonathan Brostoff. Because of the programme his waiting list had jumped to a year.

I'd already had my second child by this time. His pregnancy was much much better, only because I'd decided to take it under control myself this time. The difference was I ate a lot. Although I was pretty much as anaemic as before I was much stronger. I ate vegetables, meat and fish because I knew they were good for me. The thing is I used to have a lot of Marmite, mad keen on Marmite. I had it on toast for breakfast every day. Pure yeast, absolutely disastrous. I used to have quite a lot of yeasty things actually. I was also addicted to chocolate.

My bloated stomach got worse. I didn't get wind. I never felt there was anything wrong with my bowel. It was my stomach that was the problem. I used to get these headaches on the left side of my head which were completely associated with candida and I always had to sleep on my left side. Whenever I got a bloat I got a headache if I had something round my waist. It sounds like a joke!

My mother-in-law continued to pressurise me to go and see this allergist, Dr Lester, and my husband encouraged me as well. She had had arthritis cured. All the doctors had said that she would be crippled in the next few years. That was years ago and she's now actually better than she was. She talked to him about me and he said that he could help me. So I went along very reluctantly to him. My parents are totally anti-allergy or anything like that. They just say its all hokum. I've been brought up thinking that all that sort of thing was hokum. It was very hard to get me to go to the allergy doctor. Partly because it raises your hopes every time you go to see someone, and to have them dashed yet again. In fact that was my main reason, because I can't face going and failing again. It's so depressing. I prefer not to try.

When I told my symptoms to other doctors I felt an utter idiot. They do sound ridiculous. They just sound very odd. I think other people used to think they were pretty odd as well. But this allergy doctor didn't think they were odd at all. This was the first time that I'd come across anyone who reacted like that. He listened very carefully and asked me questions about antibiotics and things, and then diagnosed me the first time he met me. He said that he thought I had candida. He gave me some nystatin and put me on the Stone Age diet. I have no dairy products, no yeast, no grains. It's mainly meat, vegetables, fish, fruit and nuts. I felt terrific on the diet and the nystatin. I did not believe it would work at all. I had no hope at all, but after about four or six weeks it started to work.

I could tell it was actually the nystatin that was working, more than the diet, because later on when I was not having any bloats at all I started saying I don't want to take the nystatin. Six weeks of taking an antibiotic did not make me feel happy. So then I stopped taking it and within a few days it came back. I carried on with the diet. I tried that a number of times, and each time my symptoms came back. We tried substituting acidophilus for the nystatin but that was no good.

I was so keen not to have the symptoms it was hard to get myself off it. And then an amazing thing happened. I found I wasn't needing to take the nystatin. Now I've got to the point where I haven't had to take it for about six weeks. I still try to stick to the diet. I tend to feel much better if I eat a lot of fruit and vegetables.

Three years on Jessica is still well and free from problems. She recognises that her symptoms do come back if she is under stress and if, at the same time, she eats the wrong food, and doesn't get enough sleep. But although the eventual outcome is a positive one, she went through five years of exhaustion and fatigue, struggling through two pregnancies, which were undoubtedly affected by her condition, before she got better.

Can we really ascribe these problems to *Candida albicans* when most doctors are still unaware of, or deny, its wider role? The evidence from the interviews in the following chapters suggests that patient awareness is running ahead of orthodox practice. And if improvement results, is it acceptable to carry on defending the denial by ascribing recovery solely to psychological change or placebo effect?

5
WHAT CANDIDA DOES

When friends and acquaintances used to ask me what I was doing, and I told them about my interest in candidiasis, they would almost invariably reply 'Do you mean thrush?' By thrush they meant candida as it affected the mouth or the genitals. These are the most easily identifiable aspects of candida, the most popularly known, and also the only symptoms at the less chronic end of the scale to be officially recognised by doctors. Those that did know about systemic candidiasis almost invariably were informed because they knew someone who had the condition.

THRUSH

Babies often get thrush in the mouth, usually picked up by contact with candida on the journey from the womb through the vagina. It is not difficult to treat, particularly if the baby is breastfed and thus benefits from the mother's immunity. More serious, however, is the persistent presence of candida in the mouth associated with AIDS. Candida is a marker for problems of immunity. Other infections and lesions in the mouth frequently become colonised by candida, and in this way can affect people with sores from dentures, or mouth ulcers.

Most women get thrush or vaginitis at some time in their life. It causes an itchy vulva and/or vagina, and produces a thick discharge, often smelling of yeast. Candida is not the only cause, but it is the predominant one. The vagina provides a warm and moist breeding ground for candida, particularly if the normal acidity is disturbed. It is commonly treated with an antifungal cream such as nystatin, but this does not affect candida when it has become deeply embedded in the tissues. Vaginal infection with *Candida albicans* and other yeasts is often recurrent; rather than question the value of prophylactic treatment, it is sometimes easier to blame 'patient defaults' because 'left-over drugs frequently testify to poor compliance'

(*British Medical Journal*, 23 December 1978).

One of the problems for sufferers seeking treatment is that orthodox medicine does not accept that candida can be present elsewhere without producing the symptoms of thrush at the same time. Dr Patrick Kingsley, author of *Conquering Cystitis*, however, makes the observation, based on his clinical experience, that often the thrush ceases when the candidiasis becomes more systemic – the yeast changes form to burrow deeper into the tissues and cannot be detected easily by conventional tests. Conversely, Dr Kingsley is not surprised if after treatment his patients get thrush for the first time, because this is a sign that the candida war is being won; it is forced to retreat to the surface.

CYSTITIS

Another common problem for women, but not officially associated with candida, is cystitis. It is an inflammation of the bladder which causes extreme discomfort and pain. The itching and discharge in vaginal thrush sometimes affects the outer part of the urethra, leading to a wrong diagnosis of 'cystitis' or, alternatively, the bladder can be directly affected by the candida when it is systemic.

The usual assumption is that cystitis is caused by bacteria or, less frequently, by a virus. In the beginning the doctor will prescribe an antibiotic to clear it up, but if it persists a specialist will be called in for further investigations.

Dr Patrick Kingsley in his book *Conquering Cystitis* gives a full description of the orthodox approach to cystitis, before outlining his own view about the value of understanding the candida connection. Reading it gives a clear impression of the invasive and interventionist approach of conventional diagnosis when there is no effective explanatory framework. He quite fairly points out that instruments probing the bladder, looking for congenital malformations and obstructions to the free flow of urine, need to be used to rule out such causes. But the problem for the suffering woman is that the vast majority of the results of these special tests and operations will be normal. What advice then to alleviate persistent attacks of cystitis? Retaining the bacterial cause, and with only antibiotics to wield, women are told to wipe themselves from front to back after opening their bowels, and, if vaginal thrush is present, to wear loose cotton underwear.

One popular paperback, written by a gynaecologist, gives us an idea of how a section of the medical profession rationalise their 'treatments' when they fail. Dr Derek Llewellyn-Jones in *Everywoman: A Gynaecological Guide for Life* suggests that although an 'irritable bladder' is occasionally due to some disorder such as an infection, in most cases it is due to an emotional upset which shows itself in this way. Somewhere in the circular argument of cause and effect psychological factors have a place. But women find it strange that these arguments are used selectively, i.e. almost exclusively about women's health problems and not about men's!

SYMPTOMS IN SEARCH OF A CAUSE

All the people interviewed for this book came to believe that they suffered or suffer from candidiasis, and some of them discovered later that they had or have ME. Yet they were not diagnosed in the early stages of the illness by their GPs or by the consultants to whom they were referred. In a couple of interviews, the respondents spoke enviously of other sick people with high profile illnesses, such as cancer and heart disease. At least they were presenting classifiable symptoms to their doctors who could then test them and come up with reliable results. In other words the experience of being ill was not complicated by the experience of not being believed.

Candidiasis does not slot into most doctors' package of symptom clusters, partly because it is not confined to one particular organ, and partly because its discovery has still to become accepted as medical orthodoxy. The claims for candida's symptoms are very wide – digestive, nervous, cardiovascular, lymphatic, respiratory, urinary, endocrine and musculoskeletal. Doctors therefore find it difficult to drop their compartmentalised view of the body, which is not dependent on the interrelationship between organs.

Symptoms vary according to sex, from person to person, and in the same person at different times. Although diagnostic tests are being developed and used, one way for clinicians to diagnose is to rely on an understanding of each patient's clinical picture, trying to relate onset of symptoms to events which trigger yeast growth.

One way of categorising symptoms is to divide them into

those that result from direct contact with the candida along the intestinal tract and in the vagina, and those that result from the release of yeast products into the bloodstream affecting other organs. In the first category, symptoms include oral thrush, heartburn, wind, indigestion, diarrhoea, mucus or blood in the stools, constipation, colic, abdominal distension, rectal itching and haemorrhoids. In the second category there is depression (although there are sex differences here), loss of memory and concentration, weight fluctuations, loss of libido, clumsiness, vertigo, ear problems, sleeping problems, cystitis, joint pains and fungal infections of the nails and skin. Food intolerances and food allergies are also very prevalent.

Some of these symptom clusters are recognisable from other conditions, but this is no reason to accuse their owners of making overly grandiose claims. Some sufferers of ME could recognise their symptoms from this list, and they may not necessarily suffer from candida overgrowth. The slight variations, aside from individual differences of response, stem from different constellations of causes. Furthermore, different causes may, in the long run, have the same effect. It is not a question of one cause, but of many interacting forces. When looking for causes, one possibility, whenever there are pre-existing problems, is candida overgrowth.

PICKING UP CLUES

Dr C. Orian Truss first presented his data about candidiasis in *The Journal of Orthomolecular Psychiatry* in 1978, using case histories from his own practice. In that article Dr Truss argued that the presence of candida in most of us may account for the medical neglect in attempting to link this yeast to serious disease. He put forward the hypothesis that candida could move beyond the visible external symptoms and set up other symptoms throughout the body that ranged from mild to severe, affecting not only tissues and cells but also the mind. It can do this by changing from its yeast form to its fungal or mycelial form. The fungus produces root-like structures called rhizoids which can burrow through the intestinal lining. Such penetration allows toxic wastes and incompletely digested protein to enter the blood and gain circulation within the body. Thus allergic reactions, or food sensitivities, can be formed, within an overall depression of immunity and cell damage.

It is interesting that the first case which alerted Dr Truss to this possible role of candida was a woman suffering from allergic rhinitis and migraine headaches, together with severe premenstrual symptoms including vaginitis and depression. This was in 1961. Upon finding that *Candida albicans* was one of her allergens, he noticed that not only her headache, but also her depression, were relieved by injecting a small dose of candida extract.

In 1961 not many doctors were interested in the possibility of a physical basis for premenstrual problems. Women's health was not yet seen to be all that different from men's, except for the inconvenience of the monthly cycle, the interruption of pregnancy and the drying up of the menopause. Their mental health was a different matter. Many women have Dr Truss to thank for not allowing his clinical observation to be distorted by commonly accepted views of women as neurotic and hypochondriacal.

Moving from that first case, Dr Truss, and many others over the years since then, have achieved remarkable results with a wide range of symptoms and diseases, including recurrent migraines, long-standing acne, joint pain resembling arthritis, allergies, schizophrenia, multiple sclerosis, endometriosis, infertility, menstrual problems and depression. Whilst not claiming that everyone with these conditions is helped when treated for candidiasis, he is able to demonstrate that candida could be a factor, and should therefore be taken account of rather than ignored. Dr Truss attempts to describe the typical manifestations as follows:

> If we were to try in one simple sentence to describe the clinical picture most suggestive of this condition, it would be that of a woman between puberty and menopause who has been having vaginal symptoms (discharge, itching or both) and/or bowel symptoms (constipation or diarrhoea, excess 'gas', abdominal distension and discomfort), abnormalities of the menstrual cycle and flow, absent or diminished libido, and a personality change characterised by abnormal emotions (depression, extreme irritability, anxiety, crying), deterioration in intellectual function (concentration, memory, reasoning), and a destructive loss of self-confidence so severe that it may result in her inability to cope with even the simplest problem.
>
> *The Missing Diagnosis*

Although the typical case here is a woman, it should not be forgotten that men get candidiasis too. But it is essential to understand the factors that encourage candida that are specific to women.

WHY WOMEN MORE THAN MEN?

Central to the outcome of candidiasis in women, as opposed to men, is the complicating factor of hormonal fluctuations throughout the monthly cycle, and the way that candida reacts with the female hormones progesterone and oestrogen. Once candida has become chronic in women it is usual for hormone function to be disturbed. Equally, pregnancy or corticosteroid-induced hormonal imbalance (e.g. the pill) can lead to depressed cellular immunity, predisposing to candida infections.

The endocrine glands are tissues that manufacture hormones, which are released into the bloodstream to influence the physiological processes of the body. For example, the adrenal gland produces adrenaline and cortisol, the testicles produce testosterone, and thyroxine comes from the thyroid. In women the ovaries produce two main female hormones, oestrogen and progesterone, which together influence menstruation and the functioning of the uterus. Their influence is not specific to the uterus, but also important for the brain and many other tissues. Oestrogen is produced throughout the monthly cycle, whereas progesterone is at its highest level after ovulation until the following period. During pregnancy progesterone levels are consistently high.

Many women with candida problems report that their symptoms are much worse from ovulation, at the middle of the cycle, until their next period, and during pregnancy, and it has been found that progesterone, highest at these times, is directly responsible for stimulating yeast growth. Dr Luc de Schepper associates high progesterone with increased glycaemia or glucose in the blood. The commonly experienced cravings for sugar before menstruation seem to be explained by this fact; the sugar feeds the yeast, which then demands more, and subsequent depression and mood swings result from increased sugar intake.

Oestrogen-responsive tissues, including the vagina, the bladder and certain areas of the brain, are less activated when cells are compromised by candida. Thus the mental symptoms associated with candida are also encouraged by impaired hormonal response. Dr Truss points out that this association is likely because the mental symptoms are much less severe in women pre-puberty and post-menopause, and in men. Other indications are weight fluctuations and fluid retention, loss of sexual feeling and endometriosis (a condition whereby patches of tissue similar to the lining of the uterus have been found growing in parts of the body where they do not belong).

THE BIRTH CONTROL PILL

The association between hormones and candida is further confirmed by the fact that taking the birth control pill, which contains progesterone and oestrogen in varying amounts, encourages yeast growth.

Progestogens dry up vaginal secretions, and vaginal infections, including thrush, are more common amongst pill users. Vitamin and mineral deficiencies are attributed to the pill, particularly deficiencies of zinc, vitamin C, vitamin B6 and folic acid. A shortage of zinc, common in pill takers, inhibits the conversion of stored vitamin A to a usable form, so that there is a build up in the liver to toxic levels. Vitamin A is important to maintain the integrity of mucous membranes. Dr Ellen Grant, author of *The Bitter Pill*, links this shortage with a tendency in pill users to develop candidiasis. And zinc deficiency has further consequences.

> When women on very low zinc diets take oral contraceptives they enter a vicious cycle of declining health. The pill may alter the actions of the zinc and dependent enzymes in the gut lining and absorption of zinc and other minerals can be impaired – leading to further zinc deficiency and yeast or candida overgrowth releasing fungal toxins causing more allergies and reaction to carbohydrates and sugar.
>
> *The Bitter Pill*

The combination of candida-inducing effects and nutritional deficiencies, both promoted by the pill, should alert women to the dangers of oral contraception. The common practice of prescribing the pill to adolescent girls with menstrual problems, because it prevents ovulation, only makes matters worse for those susceptible to candidiasis.

Another factor that predisposes women taking the pill or steroid medication is the yeast's ability to thrive on steroids, particularly corticosterone and progesterone. When penetrating the cells looking for nourishment, the fungus is stimulated by the steroids within.

APICH SYNDROME

The acronym APICH stands for autoimmune polyendocrinopathy immune disregulation candidiasis hypersensitivity, and describes a range of disorders that can arise from the exhaustion of the immune system. The full list of problems is 26, ranging from disorders with various endocrine glands such as the thyroid and adrenals, through diabetes, pernicious anaemia and hepatitis, to premenstrual syndrome, myasthenia gravis and coeliac disease. It even covers autism and schizophrenia. While it is important to point out that these are all problems which candidiasis sufferers are prone to, and will not necessarily go down with, it is useful to look at two of the most common ailments.

If the endocrine system becomes exhausted, as it usually does in cases of candidiasis that are difficult to treat, it is likely that women go on to develop thyroiditis, which is an inflammation of the thyroid gland with an abnormal immune response in which lymphocytes invade the thyroid tissues. This is an autoimmune dysfunction. Testing for thyroiditis is difficult, but surface markers are thinning and brittle hair, rigid and brittle nails and a complexion which is pale and pasty, with puffy skin. The endocrinologist Dr Phyllis Saifer is alerted to the possibility of thyroiditis in the difficult-to-manage brittle patient with symptoms of fatigue, depression, chilling, constipation and irregular menses. Trowbridge and Walker, authors of *The Yeast Syndrome*, note that the incidence of thyroiditis in women is ten times that of men. Men are not excluded from the APICH syndrome, but the more complex nature of women's hormone balance makes it much more likely that women will predominate.

The next most common sign of endocrine exhaustion related to candidiasis is oophoritis, an inflammation of one or both ovaries in women. Dr Saifer links this condition with infection or blockage in the Fallopian tube. It may be a cause of infertility. Treated with antibiotics, this condition gets worse and, long-term, can result in hysterectomy (as can endometriosis). It is interesting that one of the interviewees noticed that after electing to have a hysterectomy her symptoms cleared for a few months, but they soon returned to concentrate on another 'target' part of her body.

Dr Edward Winger, presenting his findings at the same time as Dr Saifer (The Yeast-Human Interaction Symposium, San Francisco, 1985), endorsed her observations. He saw the problem as a triad of disorders, consisting of first candidiasis, second autoimmune antibody production and third endocrinopathy. The first line of treatment is for candidiasis.

Most of the sufferers of APICH syndrome are genetically predisposed – endocrine system exhaustion is just the final outcome of a life-long history of health problems that echo those of one or both parents. A weak capacity to defend oneself against any one of the many different strains of candida is handed down genetically from mother to daughter. This being so, it is all the more important to respond quickly to yeast problems before they become systemic and more difficult to overcome.

A second group of women candida sufferers are those that develop candida as a result of iatrogenic (doctor-caused) disease. Women are more exposed to the over-use of antibiotics because of the common recurrence of symptoms such as thrush and cystitis. Taking repeated antibiotics kills the natural flora of the gut, and allows the yeast to flourish. Taking the pill, composed as it is of artificial steroids, is also a likely contributor to women's susceptibility to candida infestation. Naturally these external triggers do not always induce problems – some women are more susceptible than others; a useful indication of possible danger is if the woman reacts badly when first taking the pill.

CANDIDA IN MEN

Although it is correct to see candidiasis as affecting mainly women, it is not easy to be clear about the size of the problem in men. When it comes to admitting illness, there are differences. Men have difficulty talking about it. Women do not have the same difficulty, and in that way have more access to information that is not available from conventional channels.

Women are practised at focusing internally. Our sexuality is not threatened by admitting to 'weakness' because that is precisely what the cultural stereotypes predict. Women are used to sharing information about health, because that has often been the only resource there is within a medical context that is dominated by male concerns.

Men do not normally have informal networks of health information, because admitting to the need for them would threaten their reliance on the image of men as strong and unassailable. Is this the reason, therefore, that one doctor, at least, has noticed that ME affects both sexes equally? In other words, is it only when an illness is so debilitating that it cannot be denied – literally when muscles can no longer support the body – that men are forced to look at how they function physically?

The literature on candida in men is sparse. Dr Truss observes that yeast growth in men is restricted to the intestinal tract and the prostate gland, but rarely found on the male genitalia. It is likely, however, that the incidence in men is higher than estimated.

The most common clue that a man may have candidiasis is prostatism – difficulty in starting to pass urine, an inability to finish completely without dribbling, and the need to pass water in small amounts frequently. If candida is the cause, it is then unnecessary to remove the prostate; but because candida is not often recognised, this operation, sometimes resulting in impotency, is usually performed.

Dr Truss claims that men who have candida do not have the same extremes of mental symptoms as women, but they do share the chronic fatigue and irritability.

OTHER SYMPTOMS

We have looked at how some of the mental symptoms produced by candida are caused, and it is clear that they are not all dependent on hormonal dysfunction.

The brain consumes 22 per cent of total blood sugar and 25 per cent of resting oxygen, making it one of the most nutrient-hungry parts of the body. As US biochemist Jeffrey Bland states, 'It requires very high levels of trace elements and vitamin-derived co-factors for function, and therefore one of the first things that happen in a state of under-nutrition is, brain chemistry is affected.'

The term 'orthomolecular psychiatry' was coined by Dr Linus Pauling, the double Nobel prizewinner, to refer to the potential for altering mental health by changing the concentrations of various substances normally present in the brain. These substances include minerals, trace elements and the amino acids which make up proteins. From this it is not difficult to conclude that if undigested protein enters the bloodstream before it has been properly broken down in the gut, the brain will be deprived of essential nutrients.

The liver is the major organ of metabolism and detoxification in the body, involved in metabolising different nutrients, synthesising blood proteins, breaking down and eliminating waste products and toxins, and secreting bile. It is also the first organ to be invaded by yeast cells, on their way to other organs such as the lungs and heart.

Many of the people suffering from candidiasis reported that they have difficulty tolerating alcohol. This is because alcohol sedates the cells in the liver that filter and detoxify the blood supply from the gut, allowing undigested foodstuffs and chemicals to escape from the liver and gain access to the general circulation. These incomplete proteins and toxic materials then affect mood, memory and behaviour, as well as produce other far-ranging systemic effects including sore joints, chest pains and skin problems. Cerebral allergy, leading to mood swings and depression, is also common.

Food intolerances are a frequent effect of candidiasis. The immune system reacts to these 'foreign' substances by treating them as antigens. Foods that would normally be tolerated become harmful and set up reactions in the brain or in localised tissues. Even if the offending foods are carefully removed from the diet, many candida sufferers find that they are merely replaced by a new list of intolerances, so that the battle is not usually won purely by avoidance alone. Thus apart from nutrient deficiency, the antigenic 'assault' on the immune system from undigested protein also has a devastating impact on the body.

Another process leading to 'brain fag' and brain dysfunction is the acetaldehyde effect; this interferes with the normal automatic functions of the autonomic nervous system, so its effects are not limited to the brain.

The anaerobic (absence of oxygen) environment of the

intestines allows the yeasts to convert sugar and digestible carbohydrates to acetaldehyde. If the liver's capacity for converting the acetaldehyde is impaired by overload or lack of the right enzyme, the following results ensue:

> Acetaldehyde binds strongly to human tissues, and, like the related substance formaldehyde, it has a significant potential to injure body organs by 'pickling' them. During moderate acetaldehyde production, the compound can bind to the cells of the intestine, liver, brain, and portal [liver] blood vessels; to their contents such as nutrients, enzymes, vitamins, polypeptides; and to the blood constituents of platelets, leukocytes, erythrocytes, and circulating proteins. During excessive acetaldehyde production, these harmful bonds can be formed throughout the body. The bonding is cumulative and quickly becomes irreversible when exposure to acetaldehyde is prolonged. Thus tissue injury as a result of polysystemic chronic candidiasis is a very real possibility. This explanation helps to make more understandable how Candida infestation can show such a broad range of symptoms, affecting virtually all body functions and symptoms . . . Many neurotransmitters are amines (derived from amino acids) and can be bound to acetaldehyde, forming 'false neurotransmitters.' Such false neurotransmitters may be the initiators of depression, anxiety, the vague uneasiness associated with stress, schizophrenic like symptoms, difficulty with concentration, and possibly lapses in memory.
>
> Trowbridge and Walker, *The Yeast Syndrome*

And so we return to the gut, the start of the journey (unless the candida has been passed on by genital or oral contact, or infection from hospital treatments). Many people report problems with bloating, excess wind, diarrhoea, constipation and abdominal pain. As we have seen in the first chapter, when candida gets out of hand other bacteria in the gut are overwhelmed and the normal process of digestion and excretion is blocked.

CANDIDA QUESTIONNAIRE

The list of symptoms is long, and not every one is discussed here. If you suspect that candida may be contributing to your health problems the following questionnaire (designed for adults, not children), devised by Dr Crook, should give you some indication of whether your suspicions are well-founded.

Section A: History

		Point score
1	Have you taken tetracylines or other antibiotics for acne for 1 month (or longer)?	35
2	Have you, at any time in your life, taken other broad-spectrum antibiotics for respiratory, urinary or other infections (for 2 months or longer, or in shorter courses 4 or more times in a 1-year period)?	35
3	Have you taken a broad-spectrum antibiotic drug – even a single course?	6
4	Have you, at any time in your life, been bothered by persistent prostatitis, vaginitis or other problems affecting your reproductive organs?	25
5	Have you been pregnant:	
	2 or more times?	5
	1 time?	3
6	Have you taken birth control pills:	
	For more than 2 years?	15
	For 6 months to 2 years?	8
7	Have you taken prednisone or other cortisone-type drugs:	
	For more than 2 weeks?	15
	For 2 weeks or less?	6
8	Does exposure to perfumes, insecticides, fabric shop odours and other chemicals provoke:	
	Moderate to severe symptoms?	20
	Mild symptoms?	5
9	Are your symptoms worse on damp, muggy days or in mouldy places?	20
10	Have you had athlete's foot, ringworm or other chronic fungus infections of the skin or nails? Have such infections been:	
	Severe or persistent?	20
	Mild to moderate?	10
11	Do you crave sugar?	10
12	Do you crave breads?	10
13	Do you crave alcoholic beverages?	10
14	Does tobacco smoke *really* bother you?	10
		Total score, section A

Section B: Major symptoms

For each of your symptoms, enter the appropriate figure in the point score column:

If a symptom is occasional or mild	score 3 points
If a symptom is frequent and/or moderately severe	score 6 points
If a symptom is severe and/or disabling	score 9 points

Add total score and record it at the end of this section

Point score

1 Fatigue or lethargy
2 Feeling of being 'drained'
3 Poor memory
4 Feeling 'spacey' or 'unreal'
5 Inability to make decisions
6 Numbness, burning or tingling
7 Insomnia
8 Muscle aches
9 Muscle weakness or paralysis
10 Pain and/or swelling in joints
11 Abdominal pain
12 Constipation
13 Diarrhoea
14 Bloating, belching or intestinal gas
15 Troublesome vaginal burning, itching or discharge
16 Prostatitis
17 Impotence
18 Loss of sexual desire or feeling
19 Endometriosis or infertility
20 Cramps and/or other menstrual irregularities
21 Premenstrual tension
22 Attacks of anxiety or crying
23 Cold hands or feet and/or chilliness
24 Shaking or irritable when hungry

Total score, section B

Section C: Other symptoms

For each of your symptoms, enter the appropriate figure in the point score column:

If a symptom is occasional or mild	score 1 point
If a symptom is frequent and/or moderately severe	score 2 points
If a symptom is severe and/or disabling	score 3 points

Add total score and record it at the end of this section.

Point score

1 Drowsiness
2 Irritability or jitteriness
3 Incoordination
4 Inability to concentrate
5 Frequent mood swings
6 Headache
7 Dizziness/loss of balance
8 Pressure above ears, feeling of head swelling
9 Tendency to bruise easily
10 Chronic rashes or itching
11 Numbness, tingling
12 Indigestion or heartburn
13 Food sensitivity or intolerance
14 Mucus in stools
15 Rectal itching
16 Dry mouth or throat
17 Rash or blisters in mouth
18 Bad breath
19 Foot, hair or body odour not relieved by washing
20 Nasal congestion or post-nasal drip
21 Nasal itching
22 Sore throat
23 Laryngitis, loss of voice
24 Cough or recurrent bronchitis
25 Pain or tightness in chest
26 Wheezing or shortness of breath
27 Urinary urgency or frequency
28 Burning on urination
29 Spots in front of eyes or erratic vision
30 Burning or tearing of eyes
31 Recurrent infections or fluid in ears
32 Ear pain or deafness

Total score, section C
Total score, section A
Total score, section B
Grand total score

The grand total score will help you and your physician decide if your health problems are yeast-connected. Scores in women will run higher as seven items in the questionnaire apply exclusively to women, while only two apply exclusively to men.

- Yeast-connected health problems are almost certainly present in women with scores over 180 and in men with scores over 140.
- Yeast-connected health problems are probably present in women with scores over 120 and in men with scores over 90.
- Yeast-connected health problems are possibly present in women with scores over 60 and in men with scores over 40.
- With scores of less than 60 in women and 40 in men, yeasts are less apt to cause health problems.

In this chapter we have mainly described symptoms ascribed to candida, referring in passing to causes. Moving from Dr Truss's pioneering work in the States we have been able to fit together many symptoms to make a coherent and explicable pattern. But although this may seem coherent and logical to those who suffer from these symptoms, and to those who gain relief once they are treated, this does not guarantee acceptance by anyone else. The next group of chapters tries to understand why.

6
ALLERGIES AND FOOD INTOLERANCE – PAVING THE WAY

It is important to look at how the new ideas about allergies were taken up, because that experience illustrates the same difficulties that were encountered in introducing the concept of candidiasis into medical practice. Food allergy, presenting the classic allergic reactions such as asthma, skin problems and nasal inflammation, is now beginning to be understood by doctors. But food intolerance, when reactions are less testable and specific, is a different matter; it is difficult to pin down, and the symptoms are many and varied. This is why it is not recognised by many doctors. The irony is that some of the pioneering doctors who did develop an understanding of the role of allergies, and the wider role of food intolerance, persist in treating allergies and intolerance as symptoms, rather than candida as a possible cause. Multiple allergies usually go when the body is brought back into balance; the temptation is to try to eliminate the allergies without first finding the deeper problem that may be causing them.

The word allergy was first used in 1906 by an Austrian physician, Clemens von Pirquet. In early textbooks allergy was defined as an excessive response to a reasonable provocation. Grass pollen, shellfish and strawberries are commonly accepted allergic substances for a small minority of people. However, any attempt to extend the range of potential allergens or intolerances by simple observation and elimination was pushed aside by the rising fashion of only believing what could be tested biochemically. Immunologists moved from the observation that some allergy reactions produced antibodies and certain lymphocytes to stipulating that any other reaction without these markers could not be an allergic one. It was then convenient to assume that the origin of these latter reactions was psychiatrically derived rather than physical.

Dr Theron Randolph, a Chicago physician and clinical scientist, was a pioneer in the field of allergy research. He observed that repeated exposure to any offending substance moves from an 'alarm' response to one of adaptation. Such adaptation forces the body to over-produce hormones such as cortisone and adrenaline, which results in an addictive relationship to the allergen. Gradually, however, the body's adaptive potential disintegrates, leading to 'exhaustion' when the addictive 'high' no longer repeats itself. In all stages of the process, abstinence produces withdrawal symptoms such as migraine and feelings of fatigue. Treatment does not depend on drugs to suppress the symptoms, but more simply on finding the substance which causes the intolerance and removing it from the environment or the diet, whilst at the same time being aware of other possible underlying causes.

In America drug companies have a huge investment in promoting the *status quo*, which is more dependent on their products than allergy treatment. They perpetuate their influence by financially supporting some of the medical journals. The result is that convincing research about allergy treatment is suppressed, and not allowed to circulate in mainstream publications. Opposition to the ideas behind clinical ecology is strong because its principles of preventive medicine and individual responsibility for health operate against the generation of income for doctors which is dependent on a sick population. Dr Robert Erdmann, an American and a psychologist by training, was stunned when he found out that his brother, a medical doctor, had had only a morning's training in nutrition. Looking for ways to educate himself nutritionally, he was forced to take some courses for veterinarians. While the practice of medicine has come to depend on people getting sick, farmers need to rely on healthy stock and fast animal growth. Nutrition is thus an essential tool for vets.

In the UK the position in relation to health and human beings is different; if allergy treatment is successful, doctors do not lose money because their potential customers are healthier. Nevertheless the real significance of allergies and food intolerance has not been widely accepted. Barbara Paterson, in her book *The Allergy Connection*, gives four reasons why.

- Clinical medicine has been moving towards treating symptoms rather than investigating causes.
- Hospital medicine has become compartmentalised, so that different symptoms are taken to different specialists, with no understanding of a possible underlying and connecting cause.
- Medical training does not include an emphasis on nutrition.
- 'Allergy' is not a recognised specialisation, and therefore does not fit into the recognised career structure.

Barbara Paterson's book is interesting because it gives a fascinating insight into the intellectual shifts that encouraged a small group of British doctors to go against their training and embrace a new way of seeing health and illness. She interviewed a number of doctors to discover how they came to see the importance of allergies. The majority of them had been deeply influenced by one man – Dr Richard Mackarness, whose book *Not All In The Mind* appeared in 1976, selling over a quarter of a million copies over the next few years. For many this was their first introduction to clinical ecology or 'environmental' medicine, whereby assessment is made of the whole person, taking into consideration diet, background, personal relationships and exposure to environmental hazards. Those doctors who were open to the new ideas were probably receptive because they had already been alerted to the problems of drug dependent medicine. All they had needed was a framework to work within.

Dr Mackarness had met Dr Randolph in 1958, and as a result had discovered the allergic nature of his own previously unexplained symptoms. He applied the theories of Dr Randolph to his psychiatric patients at Basingstoke District Hospital. Like Dr Truss and candidiasis in America, he tried unsuccessfully to make an impact on the medical establishment, this time in Britain. Talking directly to the 'patient' is not approved of, and his success with *Not All In The Mind* alienated doctors even further.

Jessica's doctor (see page 22), Dr John Lester, now retired, was one of the doctors who came into contact with these new ideas. He had already seen the need for a new approach when he became disillusioned with modern synthetic drugs and the dangers of over-use of antibiotics. His own health problems improved when he followed Dr Mackarness's advice and, after a period of apprenticeship, he started to put into practice what he had learnt. It is interesting that, although he had considerable successes using this approach, he continued to move beyond immediate answers. He became convinced that one of the possible causes of allergies was the yeast *Candida albicans*.

Dr John Mansfield was another doctor whose medical practice was changed as a result of reading Mackarness's book. He realised his medical training had placed too much emphasis on the rare and the complex, and too little on the commonplace and preventable. Yet another doctor, Dr Patrick Kingsley, visited Dr Mackarness's clinic with the intention of setting up some double-blind studies, only to realise very quickly that the rules of scientific validity did not apply when dealing with individual reactions to common foodstuffs and chemical hazards: 'My whole perception of allergy and illness changed. What I'd been semi-conscious of for some while was now finally brought out into the open.' Like Dr Mansfield, Kingsley eventually left the NHS in order to devote more time to clinical ecology, but he did so with mixed feelings. In general practice he had been able to detect problems at an early stage, but in private practice he was inevitably consulted by a high proportion of very difficult cases who had not been helped earlier on. Both Dr Mansfield and Dr Kingsley now placed great emphasis on the need to be alert for candida overgrowth in many illnesses. Dr Kingsley has built up a reputation in particular for helping many people with multiple sclerosis by testing for allergies and treating for candida.

Other doctors were alerted to the role of nutrition and allergy by personal experience of problems with food-related illnesses. Dr Jean Monro, who was a founder member of the Clinical Ecology Group, set up after Dr Mackarness's book was published, has a husband who has multiple sclerosis and two sons who are both coeliacs. The role of the McCarrison Society in introducing doctors to nutrition should also be recognised. Dr Hugh Cox went to a McCarrison Society conference in 1977 and changed his medical practice as a result. After reading Mackarness's book in 1978 he started to use exclusion and elimination diets, and in 1980 he also started using desensitisation techniques.

Although all the doctors under the clinical ecology label share a common understanding about underlying causes of ill health, they do differ in the extent to which they are prepared to move even further from their original training to embrace other skills, and utilise them in their work. Dr Cox, for example, studied acupuncture and took courses in orthopaedic medicine and homoeopathy. He also developed a technique called bio-kinesiology for examining muscle responses to allergens under the tongue, held in the hand or placed on the skin. The tests work equally well when the substance is placed in a closed phial.

However, not all the doctors who follow the principles of clinical ecology use bio-kinesiology, because it cannot be proved scientifically how it works. They place a higher importance on remaining faithful to their original training, at least when it comes to needing to know how something works before using it, even if it is harmless and even if it can be shown to work without their knowing how. Using such techniques jeopardises their attempts to influence mainstream medicine (and get private medical funding).

Dr Brostoff, who works in clinical immunology at London's Middlesex Hospital, is an important champion of food and environmental influences on health because of his position within the National Health Service. He has also been important as a source of information in the media; at least three of the interviewees in this book were first alerted to the role of allergies as a possible explanation for their problems when they saw a 'Horizon' BBC documentary in 1985 about the politics of allergy in the USA, which also featured Dr Brostoff.

Although the years since then have sometimes seen a diminution of treatment facilities for allergy in the NHS (cuts follow old prejudices rather than foster new ideas), doctors are coming round slowly to accept the limited view of allergy. But there is still widespread cynicism about food intolerance: 'Food intolerance is still regarded by the medical establishment as a "media illness", a condition conjured up to explain a number of symptoms that are psychosomatic in origin' (Liz Hunt, *The Independent*, 23 May 1989). Nevertheless, Dr Brostoff has collected much scientific evidence to strengthen his argument that allergies and food intolerance exist, often as a result of overgrowth of infectious yeast and bacteria, and increased exposure to chemical pollutants and stress.

The difficulty is that science is selective in how it is used, and we cannot always rely on those qualified to assess science to examine their outdated certainties when challenged by new hypotheses. For that we increasingly have to rely on those who directly benefit from new ways of seeing health – the sufferers themselves.

7
THE CANDIDA WAR

When I started interviewing I had no context against which to judge what I was being told. But over and over again I was struck by a dominant theme. Here was an illness that, untreated, could progress to cause major problems, but for some reason the National Health Service was ignoring it. Of course, doctors would try to help – they would settle on one group of symptoms, carry out tests, which would usually, apart from external symptoms, come back negative. Then the patient would be shown the door until she came back with another package of symptoms somewhere else in her body. Although the American healthcare system is organised differently to our own, the following account of a typical experience in the US, taken from Dr Luc de Schepper's *Candida*, illustrates what can happen:

> The symptomatology of Candidiasis is a doctor's delight! Don't misunderstand me. It is not because the diagnosis is easy, but the broad pattern of symptoms gives each specialist in the medical field the opportunity to have a crack at this disease. That is exactly what happens. Patients consult their gynaecologists for vaginal yeast infection and are prescribed antifungal cream or vaginal tablets to take as a result. The vaginal discharge seems to disappear after 5–6 days but recurs with the next menstrual cycle or right after sexual intercourse. Again, the same or maybe another local medication is prescribed. For women with the problem during intercourse, a low dosage is advised each time after intercourse. It is not fun anymore when this repeats itself over several years, and I am sure some people could even get tired of sex when it must be followed by yet another 'pill'.
>
> At some point in the story, either the gynaecologist or the patient gets tired of the situation and the focus will be shifted away to some other symptoms. There is a wide variety of choices here! Would we like to start with the

allergic symptoms and spend a couple of thousand dollars on all the different food tests which inevitably will show some positive result? With the amount of preservatives, hormones and antibiotics we put in our food, it takes a very robust immune system not to crumble under the pressure. At this point we go through our first change of diet. Swiftly we omit some ten or twenty foods in our diet with oscillating results. We feel somewhat well on some days, but a lot worse on some other days. But do not become desperate. Another allergic test a couple of months later, show some new food allergies! Again, twenty more foods are omitted from our diet and we start having problems getting our daily menu together. And, not rarely it becomes impossible to eat altogether because we react on any food intake. 'I am allergic to everything' and 'I feel the best when I do not eat' are frequent complaints heard from such patients. Thirty pounds and two thousand dollars lighter, we finally find our way to the gastroenterologist because the bloating, gas and constipation becomes just too much for the patient (and his/her partner) to take. Upper and lower GI's are often taken and usually show nothing at all but an 'irritable bowel syndrome' or 'spastic colon'. At this point, if we are lucky, some dietary advice is provided, but more likely, an anti-gas medication, laxative or anti-spasmodicum is prescribed. What a disappointment for patient and doctor when the symptoms have a tendency to aggravate. The thought that the symptoms might have something to do with our 'nerves' is thrown in the air. That suggestion may prompt our psyche to go on with our quest for the healer. I am sure most Candida patients will see the ENT specialist for postnasal drip, the arthritis specialist for their muscle and joint pains, the urologist for the urinary symptoms, but the final specialist will, inevitably, be the psychiatrist!

At this point the readers will divide into two. There will be those who will believe the sick person when she says that she has arthritic pains, sinus problems, rectal itching, heart palpitations, depression and diarrhoea. And there will be others who will say 'Such a wide range of symptoms is not possible, either because the tests that were used prove guilt (nothing was found) or symptoms did not respond to treatment. After all, there is nothing in the textbooks to point to a connection between such symptoms. There may be some misguided, populist, quasi-scientific (the ultimate insult) theory about the "yeast connection", but until the double blind tests why should we doubt the expert view?' The best irony of all is that the sentence passed will be psychiatric treatment, the only branch of medicine which does not attempt to rely on scientific tests to prove its diagnosis.

FROM THE EXTREME TO THE RIDICULOUS

New challenges to orthodoxy will stir up deep-seated protective defences against re-evaluation, particularly when long-standing professional practice is questioned. The intriguing thing in the candida story is that 'denial' contains within it a large potential for acceptance, if you ignore the major differences in approach to healing and treatment, and separate out the more generous claims for symptoms in the unorthodox approach. One of the stumbling blocks seems to be endemic throughout conventional medicine – there is an underestimation of the extent that the mind can be affected by biochemical processes (although the newly emerging specialty of psychoneuroimmunology may change this tendency). The struggles within the ME debate may lead to shifts, with major repercussions elsewhere.

It is instructive to look closely at what is scientifically acceptable within the field of mycology, the study of fungi; in other words, establish what *is* kosher. Whether this is passed on in any great detail to the medical student is another matter.

> Although superficial fungal infections are the most common in the population, their limited range and comparatively benign nature give them little prominence in medical education. Many clinicians and laboratory workers are diffident about managing fungal infections, feeling that they are intrinsically different from bacterial diseases.
>
> Speller, *Antifungal Chemotherapy*

One well thumbed textbook, into its sixth edition, has the following to say about fungi: 'Fungi, with few exceptions, are less efficient at initiating infection than bacteria and viruses, and in temperate climates the only common fungal disease in previously healthy people are superficial mycoses, especially ringworm, and vaginal or oral thrush' (Stokes and Ridgway, *Clinical Microbiology*). But our concern is not so much with previously healthy people: our concern is in examining the likelihood of candidiasis in people whose health has been compromised by any combination of antibiotics, the pill, steroids, hormonal imbalance, poor diet, chemical intolerance, or emotional stress. This textbook does not have anything to say about those particular phenomena.

F.C. Odds, in an authoritative and up-to-date review of candida research (*Candida and Candidosis*), states that candidiasis 'infects virtually every tissue of the body', with the exception of hair. It is also observed, from examples in the case literature, that sometimes patients who have been managed on the mistaken assumption that they had a candida infection in a single deep organ reveal the true disseminated nature of candidosis only at post-mortem examination. There's nothing better than cutting people up for proving that something exists!

Scientific medicine accepts that candidiasis can become chronic, particularly in mucocutaneous candidiasis (candida infection of the skin and mucous membranes), because of a defect of host resistance. Thus persistent and widespread oral, genital, skin and nail plate candidiasis can be caused by immune deficiency. Reflecting the fact that specialists only see the rare and the complicated, the examples that are given are of babies presenting with classical primary immune defects, but the specific problem encouraging candidiasis is a defect of T-cell immunity.

Where the immune defect is narrow and almost specific for candida, such cases generally present in later childhood rather than infancy. Once again the reason that they are noticed is not because of candida but because these children have other diseases such as endocrine defects, hypoparathyroidism, Addison's disease, diabetes or hypothyroidism. The possibility that such problems could sometimes be related to the undue susceptibility to yeast infections is, for most cases, discounted.

Where immunity is compromised, textbooks advise that the standard treatment of antifungal chemotherapy should be supplemented by treatment from other specialists in immunotherapy and endocrinology. Clearly, managing the patient under such circumstances is not easy. There are hints in the texts that such complex interventions do not necessarily end successfully. Furthermore, 'immune reconstruction' is not always feasible, according to the conventional view, forcing physicians to rely on anti-candida therapy alone.

Anti-candida therapy is drug treatment, but there is no safe and effective drug that can be given freely. Nystatin was the first specific antifungal drug for candidiasis, but conventional medicine has restricted its use to topical treatment only because of the view that it is toxic and insoluble. Nystatin is, however, the commonly used drug recommended by medical proponents of the 'yeast connection'.

The most effective drug, amphotericin B, is seen to be highly toxic, and can permanently damage the kidney (although some clinical ecologists play down its toxicity, preferring to use it instead of nystatin). However, whereas before there was a reluctance to use such a drug without confirmation of candidiasis, F.C. Odds assures us in *Candida and Candidosis* that 'those days are over'; although doctors still cannot confirm the diagnosis, they often use amphotericin B anyway. This is called 'blind' empirical antifungal treatment, necessary when the diagnosis cannot be confirmed microbiologically. Flucytosine has less side effects, but there is a risk of resistance developing in the fungus, especially when host susceptibility to candida requires repeated use.

Odds, under the heading 'Unorthodox treatments', chooses to discuss only lactobacillus (the friendly bacteria in the gut able to keep candida under control) and garlic. He is able to dismiss lactobacillus because none of the reports of therapeutic use approaches scientific standards of evidence for a clinical effect. He could only find one study to meet his standards, but that is not relevant because, 'it hardly provides a basis for belief that bacterial preparations may achieve cures of pathological Candida infections'. To be sure, lactobacillus on its own does not have the capacity to fight against an immune system rendered powerless by man's intervention or chronic disease. But there are other, less life-threatening instances of candidiasis which could benefit. Finding the most effective combination of bacteria needs research and development, which clearly will not be carried out if their value is speedily dismissed.

Odds may be correct to be cautious but, as with the drugs he prefers, it is overly simplistic to rely solely on one therapeutic tool. It would make more sense to look at a wide spectrum of effective interventions, used concurrently. The safety of lactobacillus suggests that it has advantages over the toxicity of chemotherapy, but no research trial will show its potential for healing when used alone without a broad package of other healing aids. Unfortunately for candida sufferers this is not scientifically tidy. If you mix things together how can you 'prove' the efficacy of each individual component? It's much easier to use what you know is effective in test tubes, even though in bodies it kills off more than you would like it to.

Garlic is the second unorthodox aid that Odds singles out, although it seems that the only reason he calls it unorthodox is because it is used *au naturelle* rather than in a synthetic form. He argues that this should be no bar to taking it as seriously as other anti-fungal drugs. (The reality, of course, is that it is.)

When looking at causes of vaginal thrush, Odds can only suggest two which are scientifically proven – pregnancy and diabetes. The use of antibiotics and oral hormonal contraceptives, and their concomitant changes in vaginal pH, are not found to be associated, although he is prepared to see that there is evidence of contributory psychological problems. Specific immune status is given as the reason why some women are more prone than others to recurrent infection. But one study, based on 100 women, showed an association between ingestion of dietary sugar and recurrent candida vulvovaginitis.* Urinary sugar levels of glucose, arabinose and ribose were elevated, and these excretion patterns correlated well with the excessive intake of dairy products, artificial sweeteners and sucrose. Eliminating excessive use of these foods brought about a dramatic reduction in the incidence and severity of candida vulvovaginitis.

So where is the agreement so optimistically alluded to? First of all, there is agreement that candida exists and that it can clearly wreak havoc, whilst at the same time remaining elusive and difficult to identify. There is agreement that it is commensal, with an ability to become pathogenic given the right conditions. There is agreement that immunity is central to host resistance, but little discussion in the conventional literature about how immunity could become compromised in the first place, when inherited factors are not all responsible. There is agreement that candida often spreads from the gut,

*Horowith, B. J. et al., *The Journal of Reproductive Medicine*, 29 (1984): 441–3.

but little reference to that fact when conventional treatment regimes are devised. There is agreement that women are more susceptible to genital infections and endocrine disorders associated with candidiasis, but little energy given by scientific medicine to find out why. Peppered throughout the otherwise rigid texts are chinks in the scientific armour – psychological explanations fill the holes when other explanations cannot be found.

Reading these texts is a bit like eavesdropping on someone else's conversation when they are talking about you in a half understood language. But it is not difficult to detect an underlying theme. Treatment is applied to a passive and unknowing recipient according to scientific frameworks that exclude all explanations which challenge the core of what is already known. For the moment the two views of candidiasis are experiencing intermittent skirmishes, with a few shots from the foothills. But war has a tendency to escalate before it abates, and there are signs that the battle will not die away.

THE WAR OF WORDS

Dr Josef Issels's cancer treatment is based on immunotherapy, aimed at raising the body's own defences rather than concentrating on the tumours alone. At the base of his theories is the view that the root of many health problems, including cancer, is an imbalance in the ecology of the gastrointestinal tract. His writings on this in 1948, and since, were for many years vilified and ignored by orthodox medicine. Penny Brohn, cofounder of the Bristol Cancer Help Centre, includes him among the other *Gentle Giants* in the title of her book as one who helped her in the process of recovery from cancer. Issels's role in the 'discovery' of the part that *Candida albicans* can play in human illness has been largely unrecognised.

Dr Truss first put forward his theories about *Candida albicans* and its potential for causing many different and varied symptoms, in opposition to the orthodox restricted role outlined above, in the *Journal of Orthomolecular Psychiatry*, originally presented at a conference in 1977. This had some impact amongst a minority of doctors already interested in allergies, nutrition and diet, but little effect on mainstream medicine. In 1983 he published a book aimed directly at the general public. *The Missing Diagnosis* claims to provide the missing piece of the jigsaw, and the cover lists the numerous conditions which could be helped.

Appealing directly to the woman in the street does not claim the attention of doctors, whose first instincts are to dismiss such efforts as commercial quackery. In the same year another American doctor, Dr William G. Crook, published his book on candida called the *The Yeast Connection*. It also made grand claims that would provoke immediate scepticism in anyone who had passed through a medical school. 'If you feel sick all over, this book could change your life!' But for many who did feel sick all over, Dr Crook and Dr Truss were able to offer a possible explanation for their health problems.

Dr Crook had also written a syndicated newspaper column on health matters, and he had an appreciation of the power of the media to spread new ideas. His zeal and enthusiasm for the discovery of candidiasis is evident in his 'special offer' to any medical practitioner in Britain, when he came here in 1988 to publicise the new edition of his book. If doctors sent him their card proving their medical credentials he guaranteed to send them back a free copy of his book. Free enterprise is not responded to with alacrity, even in Mrs Thatcher's Britain; not many doctors in this country would have heard his message, and even if they had they did not rush to respond.

In Britain, candidiasis as a diagnosis became popularly available through Leon Chaitow's book *Candida Albicans – Could Yeast be Your Problem?* In the first year of publication, 1985, it was reprinted three times. Leon Chaitow, a naturopath and an osteopath, is a prolific writer on many health topics, and a regular contributor to *Here's Health*, a monthly magazine which espouses the value of wholefood diets, good nutrition and an open-minded approach to complementary medicine. His book on candida departs from Truss and Crook in that it offers an alternative treatment to the antifungal drug, nystatin. As such, Chaitow was merely echoing other American writers on candida, such as Jeffrey Bland, director of the Linus Pauling Institute.

Dr Crook, clearly relishing his missionary role, seems to pop up everywhere. For example, one of the interviewees for this book happened to go into her college on a Saturday and, walking past a lecture theatre, stopped to listen. It was Action Against Allergy's annual conference, and Dr Crook was describing some of her symptoms. Until then she had been unable to connect them. From that point she was able to go some way towards helping herself.

A friend was sitting in a restaurant in an Indian hotel, and overheard an American doctor, the ubiquitous Dr Crook, talking about candidiasis. From this she was able to explain her partner's long-standing problems with chemical intolerance, fluctuating weight gain and excessive mood swings; his childhood in America had been permanently punctuated with steroid treatment, and his use of acrylic paint in his work aggravated whatever tolerance or intolerance he had.

Celia and Brian Wright, co-founders of the Green Farm Nutrition Centre, first heard of candidiasis when they attended a clinical ecology conference. Dr Crook was the speaker. Green Farm subsequently published a newsletter which carried articles on the importance of intestinal flora and the role of candidiasis. It was their telephone advice service that finally, after a desperate call to the Citizens Advice Bureau, pulled another interviewee back from despair at ever finding out what was wrong.

In America self-help groups abound, and AIDS consciousness has operated to publicise candida even more. By 1985 candida had taken over from allergies as the 'flavour of the year', causing some journalists to take an amusing (except for the sufferers) swipe at the indulgent self-preoccupation of its victims. The hype that trumpeted this new diagnosis in North America led some commentators to add a word of caution. 'While thousands, perhaps hundreds of thousands, of genuine cases of candidiasis can and will be verified, we can not look to this disease as the mother of all complaints and to its eradication as a panacea for all attendant ills' (M. A. Weiner, *Maximum Immunity*).

In the summer of 1985 the Practice Standards Committee of the American Academy of Allergy and Immunology (AAAI) gave their reasons for questioning the existence of chronic candidiasis. They felt that it would apply to almost all ill people some of the time, and the broad treatment programme would help most illnesses whatever the cause. (It's surprising, then, that many more doctors have not changed their advice to patients when their standard treatments do not help.) They also called for published proof that *Candida albicans* is the root cause, published proof that antifungal agents help people get better, and reliable evidence of effective diagnostic tests. They expressed concern that resistant species of yeast and other pathogenic fungi would develop because of the use of antifungal agents, and caution about side effects from oral antifungal drugs. But it has already been demonstrated that conventional medicine treats systemic candidiasis in extreme situations without confirming its presence, and with highly toxic drugs. The caution about the long-term use of oral antifungal drugs is commendable, but this is no reason to dismiss the illness *per se*.

In Britain candidiasis had still not hit the media, and it was only in 1988, in the wake of the ME coverage, that articles on candidiasis first appeared in Sunday colour supplements and women's magazines, with the notable exception of Leslie Kenton's coverage in *Harper's and Queen* in March 1986. A *Guardian* article by Jillie Collings in February 1988 gave prominence to the view of clinical ecologists, at the same time allowing a conventional response which expressed fears of disturbing an already alarmed public. But, as the case material shows, many people have the media to thank for alerting them to a relevant diagnosis which no doctor had been able to provide. New Zealand and Australia had a more open approach to candidiasis, a reflection of their greater appreciation of clinical ecology and the prevalence of ME.

In Britain the Candida Albicans advice group was started by a vitamin and mineral company, G & G Food Supplies of East Grinstead. A newspaper article ((The Independent, 13.10.87) pointed to links between the Scientology Church, G & G Food Supplies and the Candida Albicans Advice Group. Whatever the truth in such claims, and they have been denied, there is clearly a need for a self-help group with charitable status and more ability to get favourable media coverage. The backlash in the ME debate – it's all in the mind – is going to affect how candidiasis is responded to in the media.

Media coverage leads to patient awareness, which leads to demands on doctors, which leads to confusion and resistance. Two articles in the *General Practitioner* in early 1989 make interesting reading. 'Candidiasis is rising in the media' heads the article by Dr Charles Shepherd, a former GP unable to work because of ME. He clearly sees no role for candidiasis in his own ME, and is grabbing the opportunity to warn his colleagues to be on their guard. Having outlined the theory behind the new thinking, which he cautions 'is not accepted by any of the consultant microbiologists I have questioned', he states that some patients accept these explanations without question. (Since when are we encouraged to question conventional medicine?) Following this passive acceptance, according to Dr Shepherd, complicated and expensive regimes are followed. (Since when were simple, low-cost treatments advocated on the National Health?) Pseudo-scientific research carried out in the US is blamed for alternative medicine's belief that chronic misuse of antibiotics by the medical profession, with other environmental factors, has reduced our resistance to candidiasis. And, last but not least, out comes the old favourite – 'some patients, undoubtedly, claim that anti-candida treatment helps, but there must be a placebo effect occurring'.

Just in case Dr Shepherd is considered too prejudiced against alternative medicine, it is noteworthy that he shares the page with another article, 'Yeast idea is only half believable', by Dr Lindsay Pritchett, who 'keeps an open mind towards alternative medicine but wonders about candidiasis'. Her practice of 'scientific acupuncture', and her referrals to osteopaths, and the fact that she 'concedes the existence of post viral fatigue syndrome', make her jokes against the latest 'quasi-diagnosis' of candidiasis all the more plausible. If these articles mould and reflect the predominant view amongst doctors in the front-line, it is not difficult to appreciate the sense of rejection and despair that such denial induces.

8
PATTERNS OF DENIAL

As will be apparent by now, the acceptance by the medical community of candida as an organism that can cause systemic disease with wide-ranging ramifications has been slow and piecemeal, and has only occurred as a result of pressure from consumers, i.e. the unfortunate people who suffer from candidiasis, and from those that speak for them. And even today it is only a small minority of orthodox medical practitioners who will subscribe to this idea and treat these patients accordingly. That this is the case should not surprise us, though; the following examples illustrate parallel stories.

PRESSURE FROM BELOW

By 1975 around 1 million US children were diagnosed as suffering from minimal brain dysfunction (MBD), now known as hyperactivity. In the early 1960s CIBA first proposed that their amphetamine-like drug Ritalin be used for children as a treatment for behavioural problems. In fact drugs such as benzedrine had been used to control unruly children since the 1930s. Arabella Melville and Colin Johnson ask in their book *Cured to Death*, 'Are children being abused and controlled with drugs simply because school is boring?' However, they miss the point.

The Hyperactive Children's Support Group was founded in 1977 by Sally Bunday and her mother Irene Colquhoun, and since then they have helped thousands of British children and parents overcome the difficulties of hyperactivity by taking account of diet and nutritional deficiencies. It was Sally's experience with her own son (he was prescribed adult doses of addictive drugs when he was only three years old), and his instant recovery on the Feingold diet (eliminating foods containing additives) that prompted her to set up a self-help group.

Although in the twelve years since the group started some

doctors and consultants have come to accept the importance of diet and its links to childhood behaviour, often thanks to the HCSG successes with otherwise unsolved cases, the HCSG still remains, for the majority of families, the only source of information and help. Interestingly, they have noted that many children with allergies and hyperactivity have mothers who have severe PMT, allergies and *Candida albicans*.

The exposure of hyperactive children to antibiotics is frighteningly high – the worst cases that the HCSG have come across have had between 40 and 70 courses of antibiotics, some for children as young as six. Furthermore, the reports that the Support Group receive from parents desperate for help suggest that GPs are still saying that children on a good wholesome diet do not need nutritional supplements. Their own experience in the clinics that they have been forced to set up to treat hyperactive children shows that many do not improve until they are given supplements and are treated for food and chemical sensitivities, after first having been checked for candida involvement.

There are many more examples of self-help groups set up in desperate need. Many share a recognition of the value of nutrition, a previous rejection by orthodox medicine, and a determination to provide hope and help where there was none before. Amelia Nathan-Hill started Action Against Allergy because of life-long problems with her health. In the beginning the name of the organisation reflected the focus of her battle, and in one sense she has contributed to an opening up of the debate about allergy in conventional medicine. But, after years of trying to help others to discover and eliminate their allergens, she has come to recognise the role of candida and ME, and more importantly the need to understand what causes the immune system to break down. As we have seen, doctors are only now broadening their cautious view of allergy, whilst many are still blind to the role of nutrition and the centrality of immune function and environmental illness.

Self-help groups and books can push forward against the 'Do nothing' approach, by sponsoring and publicising research that in the normal course of events would not necessarily be funded. Foresight, the Association for the Promotion of Preconceptual Care, founded by Belinda Barnes to counter official apathy towards nutrition, funded a research project at the University of Surrey which found abnormally high levels of lead in the foetal brain tissue of stillborn babies. But until lead became an acceptable subject, the researchers had difficulty finding a medical journal which would publish the results.

MULTIPLE SCLEROSIS

Judy Graham was forced to write *Multiple Sclerosis* because of the lack of positive suggestions for treatment and symptom management from doctors. When she wrote the book doctors had at least arrived at the point where they were willing to diagnose, albeit without testable certainty, i.e. ahead of the situation we have with candidiasis today and about on a par with ME. Hysteria, the label applied to MS sufferers for many years, had been replaced by a diagnosis which took account of physical abnormalities. But the sentence imposed – 'nothing can be done' – strikes a familiar note today; such pessimism has only been alleviated in the recent past by the patchy orthodox acceptance of special diets and nutritional supplements, largely due to the campaigning efforts of sufferers themselves.

This early pessimism implied a real sense of powerlessness. Patients, highly motivated, if not already pulled down by the expert opinion, and unrestricted by the need to wait for rigorous testing by scientific method, were forced to find out for themselves. Judy Graham's approach did not set out to court medical approval.

> The kind of therapies listed in this book do not lend themselves to the rigorous kind of double-blind controlled trials beloved of scientists. They are not drugs, and cannot be tested as if they were. Moreover, doctors are always saying that no two cases of MS are alike. If that is so, how can they possibly bunch together 200 or 300 MS cases for a trial, and how can they possibly match them against controls? This stumbling block has always baffled me when doctors start waving their 'there is no scientific evidence' finger at me. And quite apart from anything else, many people consider it unethical to deprive the control group of a therapy which they are convinced is of benefit.

Fatigue, which comes and goes in multiple sclerosis, is not now ascribed to psychological causes alone, as it used to be.

Scientists have caught up with what the victims of the disease already knew.

CHOICES IN CHILDBIRTH

Trends in childbirth, initiated by doctors and replaced by more effective patient-led alternatives, are numerous. At one stage in the mid-1970s induced births in hospital reached the 40 per cent mark; induction took away the need to depend on nature's unsocial timing, so that medical staff could do their work during the day. The fact that it also led to many complications, a higher rate of forceps deliveries and greater need for pain relief was only taken note of when campaigning pressure groups, such as the Natural Childbirth Trust and the Association for Improvement in Maternity Services (AIMS), educated women to demand a birth more in tune with their own rhythms and their baby's needs.

The fashion for giving birth lying down still persists, even though it can be shown that the action of gravity when adopting the squatting position speeds delivery and lessens pain. In the name of 'science' obstetricians tried to prevent women taking control in this way – we were told that it was more dangerous, but the reality was that the need for the doctor to get on his/her hands and knees and cooperate with the labouring woman as an equal partner was too threatening to professional sensitivities. To be sure, many women prefer to hand over control to doctors, and therefore accept all the interventions that are available; in this sense, doctors are willing accomplices. But science is brandished as a reason to deprive women of choice – which may in the end involve safer options.

It is interesting that one hospital in the UK has been forced to give up epidural anaesthesia for childbirth, except in extreme cases of need, not because doctors recognise the complications that can ensue when women cannot feel enough in order to push, but because the financial cuts do not allow them to have enough anaesthetists on duty to administer the drug on demand. Women thus benefit not from soundly based argument, duly considered and taken on board, but from cuts in budgets which 'deprive' them of pain relief that may not be necessary in the first place if they were allowed to give birth in the most natural position.

POORLY TESTED DRUGS

In fairness, fashions in medicine cannot always be ascribed wholly to the enthusiasm of doctors. Women, eager for an easy and reliable method of contraception, asked few questions in the beginning about what the contraceptive pill would do to their bodies. The link between the drug manufacturers and the authorities invested to approve safety is clear in many examples of unsafe drug usage, only coming to light after fatalities and long-term effects make themselves apparent.

> When Enovid was approved as a contraceptive, in 1960, we were led to believe it had been tested on thousands of women in Puerto Rico. In truth, as a Senate investigation revealed in 1963, the FDA's decision to approve Enovid was based on clinical studies of only 132 women who had taken it continuously for a year or longer. Most of the other original subjects drifted in and out of the testing program and were lost to follow-up. Three young women died but were not even autopsied. The person at the FDA who got behind Enovid was a Dr. William Kessenich, then the director of the Bureau of Medicine. He apparently had persuaded FDA Commissioner George Larrick that the evidence concerning Enovid's safety was far more substantial than it really was. Then, in 1964, FDA's top physician, J. F. Sadusk, left to become vice-president of Parke Davis, a maker of oral contraceptives... So crude were the initial trials that appropriate dosage was not even established. It was discovered only after millions of women had taken Enovid that the amount of estrogen in the pills was ten times as high as is usually necessary for contraception. The dosages today are a great deal lower, a fraction of what they were.
>
> Seaman and Seaman,
> *Women and the Crisis in Sex Hormones*

The list of drugs 'tested' on humans is endless. Thalidomide was a drug supposed to relieve morning sickness in pregnant women; the consequences of taking the drug were that many babies were born with terrible abnormalities in their limbs. DES, or stilboestrol, was a synthetic oestrogen prescribed for threatened miscarriage in the 1940s and early 1950s. It wasn't until several years later that it was discovered that many girls exposed to the drug in the womb were likely to have abnormalities in the cervix and vagina, and were at greater risk of developing cancer of the vagina. But research in the 1940s with rats, before the experiments on unwitting humans were carried out, showed that both male and female rats developed breast cancer, with serious abnormalities of the spleen and sex organs.

In the 1950s gold injections were used for rheumatism, before doctors became aware of their toxicity. They are still being used. Cortisone became the next wonder drug. It too led to complications – moon face, uncontrollable body hair growth, mental problems, bone fractures due to lack of calcium, necrosis of the head of the femur and cataracts. Most importantly of all it causes the depression of the immune system with disastrous consequences, one of which is fungal overgrowth. Cortisone, and its synthetic replacement, prednisone, is still being used, although with more caution than before.

Valium, a benzodiazepine tranquilliser, is the most prescribed drug in the world, with prescriptions reaching into tens of millions. In the beginning, in the early 1960s, it was thought that it would not create dependency, that its effectiveness would not wear off with time, and that there would not be problems with withdrawal symptoms. Informed GPs, not necessarily in the majority, now restrict prescriptions, and try to find out the cause of anxiety rather than suppress it; this is because giving Valium creates addiction, does not continue to be effective, and causes terrible problems of withdrawal. According to the DHSS 25 million prescriptions for tranquillisers were given out in 1985.

Women have been in the front-line of these unofficial 'trials' of convenience for drugs such as Valium. For every benzodiazepine tranquilliser prescribed for men, three are written for women. Unfortunately, depression that may be biochemical in origin is not usually recognised. Moreover, suppressing reactions to life-events and past experiences is not a long-term solution. Professor Malcolm Lader, professor of psychopharmacology at the Institute of Psychiatry in London, carried out brain scans on 20 patients who had been taking Valium for between five and ten years. Ten showed impaired function, and five showed abnormalities such as brain shrinkage and loss of neural function.

HYPOGLYCAEMIA

Hypoglycaemia, a condition caused by low blood sugar, often seen to be a precursor to candidiasis, illustrates the power of those who are unwilling to change their view of how the body works. Many of the same processes and developments that can occur later with candida are revealed. At the same time we can see how a diagnosis, hungrily eaten up by those in need of help, whilst pointing in the right direction, is not always the total solution. Just as with hypoglycaemia, candida need not be, in the end, the final explanation. But an open mind to both conditions can sometimes bring about improvement or relief, and may lead, in the future, to a more integrated approach. For the story of hypoglycaemia I can do no better than summarise it as told by Barbara Griggs in her fascinating account of the nutrition revolution, *The Food Factor*.

The discovery of the effect of low blood sugar on health was made as a result of the research on diabetes and the use of insulin to treat it. Excessive doses of insulin caused blood sugar levels to plummet, with the result that diabetics experience weakness, dizziness, panic attacks, palpitations and depression. Similar symptoms were observed by Dr Seale Harris in his non-diabetic patients, and in 1924 he published a paper in the *Journal of the American Medical Association*, suggesting that 'hyper-insulinism' could be reproduced by eating large quantities of refined sugar or flour.

Many problems were attributed to hypoglycaemia, such as alcoholism, aggressive behaviour, slow learning at school, depression and addiction. Diagnosis was achieved with a glucose tolerance test, which involved no food intake for a period of time, followed by a challenge with sugar and subsequent hourly checks on blood sugar levels. A diet was recommended by Dr Harris which cut out all sugar, tea, coffee and alcohol, and carbohydrates were reduced. (The process of digestion converts carbohydrates into glucose.) Small and frequent high-protein meals were seen to be the most effective way to regulate the problem. The results in terms of patient improvement were sufficient to earn Dr Harris the AMA's Distinguished Service Medal in 1949.

But doctors were already losing interest in a cure that demanded fundamental changes in their patients' diets, and the arrival of the first tranquilliser, chlorpromazine, in 1952, consolidated that tendency. Also, as Barbara Griggs points out, hypoglycaemia did not involve expensive specialist input – psychiatrists were threatened the most by this do-it-yourself approach. But the publication in the early 1950s of two self-help books fuelled public interest in the illness, and further aggravated official irritation.

Confirming the common trend that doctors are more likely to change when they are ill themselves, one Florida doctor took three years to find a diagnosis for his anxiety states, tremors, lack of memory and concentration problems, going through many inappropriate diagnoses on the way, until he eventually recovered on the Harris diet. Turning his zeal into action, he gathered 600 case studies, hoping to demonstrate to his colleagues the value of this neglected diagnosis. The AMA turned him down, and subsequently pronounced in 1973 that hypoglycaemia was not relevant for the majority of those with similar symptoms.

This defensive stance unwittingly echoed new doubts about hypoglycaemia, from a different perspective. Some practitioners suggested that improvements were felt when people, by chance, were eliminating foods to which they were allergic, and the original hypoglycaemic symptoms were merely signs of withdrawal from the allergen first thing in the morning, after a night without food. Some patients, whilst feeling some improvement in their hypoglycaemic symptoms, reported that they began to feel depleted in energy, with constipation, arthritis, gout, headaches and skin disorders.

At this point in the story I can hear the delighted cries of 'I told you so' from the cynics – 'Fads are fads, and if anyone gets better, and it looks as though not many did, it's the placebo effect.' But there is a twist to the tale, and that is that the best diet for hypoglycaemia has been found to be one based on naturopathic principles – complex carbohydrates, seeds, nuts, grains and vegetables. Too much animal protein, over time, risks upsetting the acid/alkaline balance, and can lead to vitamin B deficiency and degenerative disease. This does not mean that such a diet must be adhered to for life, merely that in order to restore the body to correct functioning, along with other therapies, it may be a sensible way to eat for a while.

Moving beyond hyped claims for the instant cure, the benefit of hindsight makes it easier today to view hypoglycaemia as a contributing factor in many conditions. The lessons for candidiasis are there to be learnt. But there is still a stubborn resistance to accepting the validity of many 'new' labels. Caroline Richmond, a founder member of the Campaign Against Health Fraud, speaks for a section of medical opinion when she says:

> The illness behaviour of patients and the diagnostic behaviour of doctors are susceptible to fashion, and they are part of it. *Plus ça change, c'est la même chose.* Neurasthenia, brain fever, melancholy, the vapours, hysteria, chlorosis, hypochondria – the names emphasised that the diseases were organic. Now they have lost their organic associations and imply states of personality or mind. Will the same thing happen to hypoglycaemia, Candida albicans, total allergy syndrome, chronic Epstein-Barr virus infection, repetitive stress injury, and myalgic encephalomyelitis?
>
> Caroline Richmond, 'Myalgic encephalomyelitis, Princess Aurora and the wandering womb', *British Medical Journal*, 13 May 1989.

Fashion in medicine is undeniable. Caroline Richmond talks of patient-led demand, in terms of the symptoms they *choose* to display, implying that the substance of the condition is ephemeral and 'all in the mind'. Doctors, she seems to be suggesting, follow the fashion by obligingly coming up with a new diagnosis because they are duped into treating these fanciful illnesses, without being able to see the manipulation from the all-powerful professional patient. It seems as though this particular journalist is identifying with the pique that doctors feel when they are pushed from behind rather than leading from the front.

Arguments which deal with either/or, organic or mental, are likely to appeal to those with a simplistic view of the body, or those with a vested interest in such a division because they do not have the skills to take a more holistic view. Illnesses, mental and physical, can have organic causes and effects which may require organic treatment. They may also be initiated or exacerbated, in part or in whole, by emotional stress. They can be further exacerbated by one-sided medical prejudice in favour of the 'mental' or 'physical' polarity, and positively harmed by corresponding inadequate treatment.

Fashion is usually dictated by those with powerful interests in particular trends. It is surely not correct to see that power vested only in the patient. Self-help groups arise after their particular need has been unrecognised or inappropriately treated, because of 'fashions' in medicine which become outmoded.

9
ME IN THE MEDIA

> Symptoms of ME include dizzy spells, exhaustion, amnesia and a leaky radiator in the Porsche. (*Options* magazine, November 1988)

Myalgic encephalomyelitis (ME, also known as post-viral fatigue syndrome, and chronic fatigue syndrome in USA) is a syndrome or collection of symptoms which result, it is thought, from viral infection of acute or insidious onset. Until the 1980s it was not officially recognised, with the result that many chronic cases of ME were inappropriately treated. And this is still the case for those sufferers whose doctors persist in holding on to the outdated idea of labelling the disease a psychiatric disorder. However, the self-help groups and the media have all helped to increase awareness within both medical and lay consciousness. Because it was first observed in epidemic outbreaks, it was not thought to occur in individual and isolated cases. The later assessment of the 1955 outbreak of ME in the Royal Free Hospital (292 members of the medical staff and 12 patients were affected), in which two psychiatrists concluded that 'mass hysteria' was the cause, ignored the series of sporadic cases in the same geographical area, both before and after the outbreak in the hospital. Subsequent knowledge of this syndrome was affected by lack of scientific evidence of cause, followed by failure to appreciate the scientific evidence when it did become available, and the ease with which 'unknown' illnesses can be conveniently assigned to psychiatry.

This chapter looks at what ME is, before examining the role of the media in publicising ME, the gradual recognition of ME within conventional medicine as a result of media coverage and self-help pressure, and the continued denial of the candida connection, despite evidence of candida involvement in some ME cases.

TERMINOLOGY

Naming an illness can increase its severity. Many research projects demonstrate that pain relief needs to be increased when patients learn that what they thought was a minor problem is actually more serious. But with ME the situation was different: sufferers knew they had a serious problem before anyone could name it. Part of their anxiety was alleviated once they had a diagnosis to work with.

ME used to be known as, or grouped with, post viral fatigue syndrome. They are no longer considered to be the same thing. Dr Lloyd and colleagues argued in *The Lancet* in June 1988 that ME is not solely triggered by viral involvement – other infections, including brucellosis and toxoplasmosis, and immunisations such as tetanus, typhoid, influenza and cholera, can all play a part. This is a clear indication that underlying all 'triggers', whatever they are, is the body's ability or inability to resist them.

Many of the doctors who treat allergy and environmental illness prefer to see ME in terms of overload – the body can tolerate so much stress from whatever source, but at some point the bucket gets full. Mechanisms for adapting cannot always prevent the overflow of symptoms which signal distress.

Dr A. M. Ramsay, involved in fighting for the recognition of ME since the Royal Free outbreak, points out that post-viral fatigue syndrome is more accurately applied to symptoms that clear up from a few weeks to a few months after the initial infection. At the time of writing (1989), 97 of the nurses affected by ME in the Royal Free epidemic in 1955 are still unwell, and most people with ME have a 25–30 per cent chance of still being ill after five years.

SYMPTOMS

In *ME: How To Live With It*, Ann Macintyre characterises ME by:

- Gross abnormal muscle fatigue, which occurs after a relatively small effort and from which the patient may take days to recover. This is quite unlike any fatigue ever experienced before.
- A variety of neurological (encephalitic) symptoms, most

prominent being loss of ability to concentrate, impaired memory and disturbances of sensation.
- Unpredictable variation in severity of symptoms from week to week, day to day, even hour by hour.
- A tendency for the disease to become chronic over many months or years.

The exhaustion, muscle weakness and muscle tenderness produce varying degrees of physical disability which prevent sufferers from completing the simplest of tasks. Sometimes there are symptoms of flu, including nausea, fever, shivering, aching joints, depression and headaches.

Some psychiatrists and doctors respond to symptoms of persistent fatigue and muscle weakness by recommending gentle graded exercise as a way of bringing back into use wasted muscles. Such a recommendation totally ignores all the evidence which shows that such an approach can intensify muscle fatigue. The difficulty is that it is not possible to tell whether those for whom exercise has been successful have in fact been suffering from the ME syndrome, or rather the milder version of post-viral fatigue syndrome. My experience with the interviews is that when ME sufferers come up against a doctor who recommends treatment which is totally inappropriate, such as gentle graded exercise (when in the past sufferers had already learnt that it merely made them worse), they decline to take up the offer, thus excluding themselves from the statistics of assessment and evaluation.

The brain fatigue is similar to that described in candidiasis, with often an inability to find the correct word, muddled speech and heightened sensitivity to hearing and smell. Emotions are unstable, with sudden mood changes, which were not necessarily part of the sufferer's personality before onset. Although with ME it is possible that brain symptoms may result from viral interference with brain cells, it is likely that the brain is also affected, in those cases with co-existing candidiasis, by the acetaldehyde effect and the presence of undigested protein in the bloodstream. The three to one ratio of women to men in ME parallels the higher incidence of candidiasis in women.

Digestive upsets are often experienced, and the associated frequency of food intolerance. Uncomfortable or frequent urination is common; in this context it is interesting to note that prostatism is a prime indicator of candida in men.

Temperature regulation is poor, and often the ME sufferer has cold extremities, whatever the weather. Heart palpitations and difficulty in breathing can also be present.

Clearly, those whose immune systems are compromised by emotional or environmental stress are most at risk. In terms of recovery, it is relevant that in the Royal Free outbreak the majority of the long-term sufferers were staff rather than patients; patients were resting in bed, whereas staff were forced by the nature of their jobs to carry on working, despite feeling ill. It has since been found that those who rest at the beginning have a better chance of normal recovery than those who soldier on. But because ME is only just beginning to be recognised, and does not feature in many textbooks, many people were not warned of the dangers of trying, against everything their bodies told them, to resume a normal life.

As with candida, ME is characterised by the variety of symptoms and a difficulty in finding definitive tests. Extreme fatigue cannot be measured, and doctors have to rely on the patient's testimony. But it is possible to list the most likely symptoms and diagnose from a clinical history.

Some attempts are being made to prove that ME has an organic source. Dr Peter Behan in Glasgow has found that ME can be triggered by many different viruses, and that although B cells appear normal, they are lacking in a particular surface chemical. Most important of all he has found significantly raised levels of interleukin-1 beta in ME sufferers. This chemical messenger of the immune system is known to:

- Turn on the production of other chemical messengers.
- Trigger fever.
- Act on the liver to displace protein production.
- Affect sugar metabolism.
- Break down cartilage and increase break down of muscle.
- Act on the nerve and muscle cells.
- Cause sleepiness and appetite loss.
- Decrease white cell count.

Clearly interleukin-1 beta could be the cause of many ME symptoms.

The absence of a reliable test for ME, and the classification of symptoms such as headaches, malaise, dizziness, back pain and depression as 'subjective', has made it easier for orthodox medicine to overlook an organic basis for the illness, particularly before the recent media coverage and the new research results. But the psychological label has been legitimated by only one particular piece of research. In 1970 two psychiatrists at the Middlesex Hospital in London, McEvedy and Beard, reassessed some of the case histories of those involved in the Royal Free epidemic in the 1950s. They came to the conclusion that it had been an outbreak of mass hysteria, despite the objective signs of infection and the involvement of the central nervous system, and despite the fact that some of the victims were still disabled 15 years later. Some had committed suicide.

The reasons for this conclusion were that the majority of those who became ill were young women, some of whom were socially segregated (as nurses) and thus presumed to be in a suggestible state. Because no organic cause could be found, they assumed the cause was psychological, explaining some of the symptoms in terms of anxiety and hyperventilation.

In a generous mood we might forgive these men for being so influenced by prevailing images of women at the time, when such images were only just beginning to be questioned. But in 1988 Dr Colin McEvedy appeared on a BBC 'Horizon' programme 'Believe ME', defending his thesis. It was not just that history had passed him by; it was not just that he represented some of the more reprehensible aspects of psychiatry; he had painted himself into a corner because of his fear of losing face professionally. Or does he really still believe something so patently ridiculous? The problem is that the effects of that article in 1970, in terms of how doctors diagnose ME symptoms, have lasted up to the present day, with disastrous consequences for sufferers and their families.

In the middle of writing this chapter I was introduced to a neurologist, a friend of a friend. She had taken up medicine late and had progressed very quickly to a senior position. Upon hearing of the subject matter of my book, she proceeded to tell me that of course ME did not exist, that it was instead a collection of different symptom clusters, and that it was all to do with depression, without any neurological basis. Treatment for the fatigue should be gentle graded exercise because the muscle pain was merely lactic acid build-up from lack of use. She held on to the ill-informed opinion that there was no involvement of the central nervous system and felt that, because getting over a viral infection was usually quick for most of us, the fact that it wasn't for ME victims should confirm the psychological component. She was clearly a very good and caring doctor, stressing the need for a full history and a thorough examination to rule out a physical basis for the problem.

When I asked her about the Royal Free outbreak of ME in 1955 – there are still some original sufferers in wheelchairs – her reply was that some people have a need to be dependent. In her opinion, the doctor who has championed their cause over the years, Dr Ramsay, made up the diagnosis in order to advance his own career. (A more accurate assessment would be that his courage in going against his colleagues prevented him from becoming a professor.)

This casual conversation does not necessarily represent the views of the majority of neurologists, but it does throw interesting light on the process by which new illnesses are classified as psychological until convincing evidence to the contrary overcomes entrenched orthodoxy.

ACCEPTED WISDOM

The 'mass hysteria' thesis was taken up unquestioningly by the popular press at the time, and has informed medical reaction up to the present day. Thus, for example, a textbook published in 1987, *Organic Psychiatry: The Psychological Consequences of Cerebral Disorder*, ignores both the reasoned response of the minority arguing against the 'mass hysteria' verdict, and the fact that McEvedy and Beard's re-examination of the disease was merely on the basis of some atypical cases from the time, rather than from examining people still ill 15 years later. Admitting that the situation is unresolved, the text nevertheless concludes that future epidemics will need to be carefully scrutinised with McEvedy and Beard's hypothesis in mind.

How, you may ask, can a diagnosis of mass hysteria apply to the vast numbers of individuals experiencing ME? The fact that it was epidemics that brought doctors in touch with this illness has obscured the equally relevant fact that it is not confined to epidemics. Perhaps it is because individuals can be ignored and large numbers cannot.

THE MEDIA

But the situation is changing. So much so that there is,

paradoxically, a contrast in Britain today between the public awareness of ME and the lack of popular familiarity with the candida syndrome, despite the fact that there are many similarities between the two conditions. When people asked me about my book, I knew from experience not to expect a glimmer of recognition when I mentioned candida. Instead I learnt to say 'an illness that doctors don't recognise'. In nearly every case, the reply would always be 'Is it ME?' It is interesting that whilst the medical profession continue to ignore the full significance of allergies and environmental illness, they have failed to escape the avalanche of patients clamouring for help with ME.

Sue Finlay's article in the *Observer* Weekend section (1 June 1986) must take some credit for this. She described her experiences with ME, and how she first felt signs of recovery when she was treated for candida. In the following few days 14,000 readers applied for the factsheet. From that article the ME Action Campaign was established, aiming to complement the other self-help ME group, the ME Association. The latter, founded in 1976, is primarily concerned with support, counselling and research within a conventional framework. This cautious approach may be the outcome of their early difficulties when trying to change medical opinion in the late 1970s. The ME Action Campaign, with a fresh start, developed a more openly aggressive campaigning style, capitalising on the stories and press coverage of well-known ME sufferers like Clare Francis.

The public was already being exposed to the dangers of mystery viruses – AIDS and the HIV virus, we were led to believe, were spreading at a frightening rate, and here was ME, a viral illness that didn't depend on sexual or blood contact. Enormous sums of money were being poured into the search for an AIDS vaccine: ME sufferers couldn't even get a diagnosis from their GP.

Sue Finlay's MP happened to be Jimmy Hood, the Labour member for Clydedale. He was curious to find out what name belonged to a voice on his answering machine – a woman was asking for help with an illness that he had never heard of. The illness clearly involved extreme fatigue because before the caller could finish the message her voice trailed off into nothingness. A few months later Sue Finlay called back, and from that initial contact a Private Member's Bill was sponsored by Jimmy Hood in 1988. No other disease has had to take the drastic step of getting statutory recognition in order to gain medical recognition. The Bill was never introduced because time ran out in that session in Parliament, but the House did vote in favour of hearing the Bill.

The media saturation of ME stories, and the seemingly unending books appearing on ME, have given rise to the defensive cry of 'fashionable disease' from those caught unawares, forced to consider their patient's self-diagnosis from the latest colour supplement article.

Many of the people interviewed for the media were later accused of being successful and middle class – hence the attribution of broken down Porsches to the ME symptomatology. The irony is that using high-profile cases brought the attention of the public and the medical profession to bear on this 'new' illness, and helped the plight of the many others who came from different social class groups, who had previously been ignored or who had readily accepted their symptoms as part of the social context of their lives. There may indeed be a particular personality who succumbs to ME – high achievers predominating, and those who push themselves when they initially get ill rather than rest. However, this is speculative, and ignores the many thousands who do not fit into this category.

Using the media was an effective way to seek out other sufferers. But to be fair, the media did not have to be wooed; the stories of adults and children whose lives were paralysed by extreme fatigue, muscle weakness and food intolerance made good copy. Children unable to go to school, branded as school phobic and taken by force to psychiatric hospital wards in order to break them from what was seen to be their parents' neurotic grip, made the headlines with ease because of the shocking fact, denied by psychiatrists, that they were suffering from ME rather than excessive mother love (*The Independent*, 18 June 1988).

REARGUARD ACTION

But the backlash was already there. The media began to pick up on the research from the Charing Cross Hospital on hyperventilation, which sought to show that patients with 'a presumptive diagnosis of ME' were found instead to be suffering from exhaustion and hyperventilation. The following extract from an article in *Social Work Today* (10 March 1988) represents the views of many who came to view ME as 'yuppie flu':

> Am I being excessively unkind when I wonder if the newly-discovered myalgic encephalomyelitis (post-viral fatigue syndrome or ME) has definite middle-class overtones? Somehow, it doesn't sound like arthritis or halitosis – honest, down-to-earth ailments. It has to me the same sort of ring as dyslexia, which I always think conjugates rather well. My child has dyslexia, yours is a slow learner, hers is as thick as two short planks.
>
> The same with ME – I have ME, you are rundown, she really ought to pull herself together.

The author, Judith Oliver, has every reason to be sympathetic to the plight of those incapacitated by illness – she founded the Association of Carers, an organisation concerned with the difficulties of carers of the disabled and infirm. The extension of the mobility allowance and sickness benefit to ME sufferers must have seemed too big a slice of the cake when, with the other hand, the government were reducing the help that they were giving to those who were already disabled.

Miriam Stoppard also joined the sceptics in a Yorkshire TV programme broadcast in June 1988. Tony Harbron, an ME sufferer, complained to the Broadcasting Complaints Commission that the programme was inaccurate and unfair in putting forward the view that ME was not a genuine organic illness, and that sufferers were malingerers. The complaint was not upheld, but it is nevertheless interesting to read the evidence presented by the medical adviser to the programme, Dr Tony Smith, also the deputy editor of the *British Medical Journal.* Within it we come across a familiar stumbling block – the acceptance that ME is genuine, with 'real' symptoms, but the attribution of those symptoms to psychological causes, without an acknowledgment of the organic base as well. He stressed the need for early diagnosis in order to prevent patients 'who believe they have ME from becoming trapped in a state of psychological invalidism'. Candida, allergy and hyperventilation ('ill-defined disorders') are taken up by some sufferers, Dr Smith alleged, as causes of their ill-health when in fact they are unwilling to face their chronic psychological disorders.

Dr Smith's views are repeated with alarming consistency in the pages of the *British Medical Journal* and other 'trade journals'. Buried beneath the standard formulae of scientific argument, which politely pretend to reasonable debate, are certain core judgments that have yet to be proved with the same rigour that is expected of 'the other side'. All statements are prefaced by the admission that ME is real, but this is then followed by pleas from rebuffed psychiatrists that they should be in on the act. Simon Wessely, writing in the BMJ in June 1989, was disturbed by the repeated theme that ME is a genuine illness whereas psychiatric disorders are not. Some ME sufferers may indeed recoil from the psychiatric solution, but if they do it is because their physical symptoms are ignored, or treated by psychiatrists inappropriately (gentle graded exercise).

THE CANDIDA CONNECTION

As you would expect, if the organic basis of ME is ignored, candidiasis is not officially recognised as being part of the ME syndrome. Indeed the medical adviser to the ME Association, Dr David Smith, is of the opinion that it is not. This is because he holds the conventional view of the role of candida:

> To my certain knowledge there has been no evidence that one can find either Candida or any kind of 'break down product' that is poisoning the system or the body's 'defence mechanisms' in Post Viral Syndrome or any types of ME. I appreciate that the prolonged use of antibiotics, the contraceptive pill, etc. can cause Candida problems, but as far as I am aware they are not associated with ME. Whether or not people with ME get a lot of antibiotics at the beginning is immaterial. I cannot see that there is any evidence that these types of problems are associated with Candida.
>
> *ME Association Newsletter,* Summer 1988

If ME sufferers claim that they have been helped by anti-candida treatment, Dr Smith accepts their progress but attributes it merely to the use of nystatin, or the particular diet, rather than the control of candida itself.

Dr Charles Shepherd, vice-president of the ME Association, in his book *Living with ME*, describes the open-minded scepticism and outright hostility of his colleagues towards the claims of candidiasis. He warns that patient requests to GPs for the prescription-only drug nystatin may only reinforce the mistaken view that ME isn't a real disease. Those of us on the other side of the fence are left wondering if doctors can so easily take a blinkered view of ME, might they not equally be mistaken when it comes to other new theories about the role of candida in other situations?

The ME Action Campaign has always recognised the possible role that candida can play in many cases of ME. It estimates that around 50 per cent of ME sufferers have problems with candida. And the Australian and New Zealand ME Society (ANZYMES), used to make a distinction between recent and long-term sufferers of ME, using their response to nystatin as a gauge of possible candida involvement. Recent sufferers did not significantly benefit from nystatin, and consequently were not thought to be affected by candida, but 50 per cent of long-term sufferers made significant improvements. ANZYMES now recognises that treating suspected candidiasis with nystatin, and diagnosing by result, may not be a reliable way to assess candida involvement, because doctors treating people with candida problems often see results with other anti-fungals when nystatin has failed, or has been of limited success. ANZYMES concludes that until more doctors acquire skills in the use of powerful anti-fungal drugs, and are able to help and support patients along this difficult path, they must rely on their own efforts to increase awareness of all the issues involved. (*Meeting Place*, Summer/Winter, 1987–88.)

Jacqueline Steincamp sees candida as one more factor in the overload hypothesis. Leon Chaitow, the most effective publicist of candidiasis in Britain, and Simon Martin, in their book *A World Without AIDS*, go so far as to suggest that viral infections may progress to ME in some people rather than others when there is a pre-existing candida problem, because an active fungal overgrowth enhances the viral activity and diminishes the ability of the immune system to defend against it. In this respect they link ME to AIDS because they both involve viral activity and incompetent immune function. The further link between the two is candida. Not everyone with HIV virus develops AIDS, just as in ME only some viral infections linger to become a problem.

Chaitow and Martin also suggest that candida affects most

if not all ME patients. Persistent viral presence is difficult to treat. Therefore they argue that it makes sense for ME sufferers to start on an anti-candida programme (although they do not recommend the use of nystatin as part of that programme).

LESSONS TO LEARN

The case studies in this book confirm the role of psychology and the need to reassess deep-seated emotional patterns as part of a wider aim to eliminate all stresses from within and without. This should include an attempt to boost immunity on all fronts, including anti-candida treatment where indicated. The case studies also confirm that opening up and exposing our vulnerability to psychiatrists who do not acknowledge the need for other treatments, except gentle graded exercise and better breathing, is not a tempting offer. Trust between doctor/psychiatrist and patient is not possible in the present climate of conventional resistance to 'alternative views', some of which offer a genuine remission of some symptoms, given the active involvement of sufferers in their own healing process.

Classifying ME as a collection of diseases and syndromes with many causes, in order to concentrate more specifically on the psychological component as a discrete entity, is one more tactic in the fruitless exercise of wrangling over 'cause'. Warning fellow clinicians about patient access to new ideas about ME in the *British Medical Journal* (3 June 1989), Simon Wessely poses this multi-causal hypothesis as a point of departure from the ME evangelists. Far from being heretical, he is following their lead.

The point of departure comes much more tellingly over treatment. Here he is forced to admit defeat, holding out for psychiatric treatment if all else fails (as it usually does within the restricted perspective) before a natural remission, in some cases many years later. As usual, the fact that conventional medicine cannot offer anything does not generate self-doubt or an open mind to new perspectives; it merely leads to suspicion, denial and defensive accusations of 'all in the mind'.

If candida is swept under the carpet, along with other perspectives for treatment outside the hyperventilation, gentle graded exercise and bed rest trio, some sufferers desperate enough not to be intimidated by 'expert' opinion can be relied on to lift up the corner.

10
CANDIDA AND ME: WORKING IN PARTNERSHIP

Despite the evidence, the controversy about candida and its role in ME continues. The following case study was recorded in 1987, one week after Karen had finally been given a diagnosis of ME. Before this she had also been diagnosed by an NHS allergy clinic as having candidiasis. In 1987 she had been ill for seven years, since she was 18. Throughout she had been looked after at home by her parents.

KAREN

Karen's problems seemed to start in 1980 when she caught flu. It was followed a month later by panic attacks and depression, causing her to fear being left on her own. At the time she was living at home, doing her exams at a secretarial college. Tests for glandular fever proved negative, so she was prescribed Valium, subsequently changed to Librium.

> All it was doing was covering up the illness. But it covered it well enough for me to continue going to work. Every two or three months I'd come down with something that looked like another flu or gastroenteritis or something. I just carried on going to work, feeling dreadful, coming home and going to bed because I felt dreadful, that's how ill I felt. Getting up the next morning and sleeping on the floor in my lunch hours. I just went on like that until I got myself off the Librium.

Her GP referred her to a behaviour therapy unit because he thought she was becoming agoraphobic.

> These behaviour therapy people said things like, try and

walk into town and mark on a scale of 0–10 how terrified you were on the way. What sort of good is that? This is what they think is helping people. I kept saying 'Nothing happened in my childhood. I am not loony. I feel ill. There's something inside me that is physically ill.'

In about August '84 people said, 'You look ill, there's no way you should be at work.' I was grey. I'd put on an awful lot of weight, and then started losing a hell of a lot of weight. In the end at work I just keeled over. Couldn't take another step. They sent me home.

Karen rested at home in bed unable to move. Then she heard about a new NHS allergy clinic nearby and persuaded her doctor to refer her there. 'I wanted to try everything, acupuncture, homoeopathy, everything. I wanted to go through the lot, and was going to start with the new clinic.'

At that time she lived on toast all day, with constant cups of tea. She was told to give up bread and dairy products.

After four days I had such a craving for biscuits and sponge. I went through a whole packet of Jaffa Cakes. So I lay off it for another two weeks. On the Saturday morning I had a small piece of brown bread toasted with jam. Delicious! I went into town an hour later and I had this panic attack. It hadn't struck me that I hadn't had one in the last two weeks. It just went right through me in the middle of town. Dad said it could be the bread. And I said no, it was just a coincidence. Then I had a bread roll for tea and by Monday I couldn't even walk. I was so weak I was in bed for a fortnight. I couldn't even move and I was depressed. The doctor said that it was a major allergy, and that nobody ever has just one allergy. Everything I tried I was allergic to. I began to think that it must be in my head. But my mum would dish something up with something in that I didn't know and I'd react.

Giving up foods and then reintroducing them induced asthma attacks.

I used to go up to the medical room at work when I had these funny states. And they thought perhaps there was something in these allergy things. Because they didn't believe it till then. I was so bad some days they had to send me home. They couldn't contain me. I'd never had asthma attacks before.

Eventually her doctor at the allergy clinic suggested that she might have candida. He prescribed nystatin.

> I was OK for six weeks – I even had the energy to redecorate my bedroom. I couldn't believe the energy. That was in August '86. Then I became suicidal again. My doctor was on holiday, so I contacted Dr Gwynn Davies, who had treated an aunt successfully. He was too far to go to, but he told me to stop the nystatin and referred me to Dr Harry Howell.

By this time she had given up trying to go to work, and registered for social security so that she could concentrate more on getting to the bottom of what was wrong with her.

Dr Howell gave her a glucose tolerance test which showed that she had hypoglycaemia. She was also put on an anti-candida diet.

> Within three weeks the depression of six years just vanished. I couldn't believe it. The other thing was that my immune system had absolutely packed up. I went back to see him about a month later and he said that he'd never seen anybody improve so much in four weeks. I was feeling so much better. I was eating potatoes, fish and vegetables, and cooking with a lot of olive oil.

Instead of nystatin, she was given thymus gland concentrate and homoeopathic candida tablets.

> I was quite rough on those for a few days but once I persevered it got a bit better. I kept improving until we got to the stage where he said, 'OK, I think you ought to have a colonic irrigation.'

The colonics removed large quantities of dead candida.

> They obviously did me good in getting rid of the candida, but as for my general wellbeing, I felt awful. After the third colonic he put in two implants of herbs and acidophilus. He said that I should start to introduce some new foods, and see how it goes. I'm now eating everything and not getting a reaction.

Despite the benefits of her treatment, Karen did not go back for further help for her remaining symptoms of fatigue. She tried returning to work part-time for two or three half-days a week, but failed to cope and gave it up.

Karen first read about ME in June 1986 when Sue Finlay wrote about it in the *Observer*. Her GP arranged for her to see the consultant physician from the John Radcliffe Hospital in Oxford, John Leddingham.

> I had a 15 minute appointment and I was in there an hour. He wrote down five pages of notes, and gave me a thorough physical examination. First of all he said 'You've had ME. Do you know anything about it?' So I said yes. He said that he was very pleased with me because I had done as much as any specialist could tell me to. I'd done the allergy side, and he was glad that I had got rid of the candida because that was an abnormal amount to have, but he said don't do it again.
>
> He was thrilled that I had done all the right things, which boosted me quite a bit. Now he says that, because I've had it for seven years, for the first few years it obviously wasn't as bad, but because it wasn't diagnosed and I didn't get the rest, it's worse now. Most people have it for less than 10 years, so it could be gone in the foreseeable future. On the other hand I could still have it in five years because I haven't rested.

Karen finds her GP very supportive.

> I'm already a member of the ME Association and my GP, she said, 'Anything you think would be best for me to read, bring it and I'll read it.' She admitted that she knew absolutely nothing. When I first came down with the allergies, she even wrote to the shrinks and said that my neurosis was caused by food. How many other people would bother to do that?

Although her candida appeared to be under control, her ME was still chronic. Overdoing things, like taking a bike ride, set her back, causing her ME to get worse and forcing her to stay at home from work.

Karen said that the only problem that she had before ME was severe period pains since she was 12 years old.

> My mother gets her periods exactly the same. So they just say that it is hormonal. I pass out with the pain, that's how bad it is. Men don't believe me when I tell them. I can't walk. I was on the pill for a couple of years to try and control my

> periods but I didn't react well so I stopped. As a child I got a lot of earaches. I've always had sore throats. Colds. That's all I ever used to catch.

Two years after this interview was recorded, Karen feels she is much calmer and more contented, attributing this change to the confirmation of her ME diagnosis. This is not because she is comfortable with such a diagnosis, merely that she feels reassured that her symptoms are, amongst some doctors, medically recognised and not all perceived as being psychologically derived. She feels that it is this shift in attitude that has helped more than anything.

She is getting no specialist help with her ME, but she does have one friend with ME who is doing gentle graded exercise, combined with psychotherapy. However Karen feels treatment based on exercise would not be appropriate for her. Her friend's symptoms were mostly to do with brain function, whereas her own have left her brain less affected, whilst attacking the rest of her body and her muscles. Her ME was acute in its onset, while her friend's ME was insidious and gradual.

Karen is now on invalidity benefit. Although she is not receiving any money from her employers, which would invalidate her benefit, she does work for them by typing manuscripts at home whenever she feels well enough. Her ME symptoms still persist, but she has retained her ability to eat most foods, with the exception of grains. She seems to suffer many flu-like viral infections in the winter months.

11
STAGE BY STAGE

We are told that science is cool, objective and impartial. Interviewing people in a way that allows them to feel safe to reveal themselves is not.

There is no denying that my interest was therapeutic for those I interviewed when they were in the middle of their illness. I did not have the responsibility of trying to help or cure. Usually we met on home ground. And usually the interview was terminated at the right moment for us both – no one was waiting outside the door for the next appointment.

The interviewees divide into three groups, some moving from one group to the other over time. Those in the first group were 'stuck', having moved beyond conventional solutions, and having tried various alternative options without success. They did not have an optimistic view of the future. For some, moving forward needed nothing more than a realistic acceptance of their condition. For others, there seemed to be underlying problems, such as malabsorption or chemical intolerance, that left no room for anything beyond sheer survival. By the time I came to write the book, those in the first group were in a minority. A few used the interview to reassess their present position and, hearing their own voices, allowed themselves to change direction or start to induce change, when they had been unable to before.

Another group had made a shift in the way they saw themselves and their illness, and the process by which they could get better. Sometimes the shift had come in a moment of crisis and rock-bottom despair, and sometimes it came as a slow realisation, after a long process of trying to find a 'cure' which could be handed out by someone else. The desperation of the former and the disillusion of the latter produced the same effect; a realisation that recovery and healing had to come from within, and that personal power and will were as important as 'expert' interventions. Along with this acknowledgment of responsibility and active participation came a recognition of the need for acceptance on all levels. This group had not necessarily got over all their symptoms, but they had the certainty that they would get over most of them, and did not expect miracles for instant recovery. For many, their problems had been developing and growing for a long time. It would be unrealistic to expect a sudden reversal.

A third group were no longer involved with their former symptoms because the problems had receded into the background so much that they could get on with their lives unimpeded.

Although men and women share various problems and strategies for recovery, I have not attempted to analyse them together because of the complicating fact of female physiology. Altogether I interviewed seventeen women and four men. The women fell evenly into two groups – those who had been through pregnancy and parenthood, and those who had not.

Pregnancy and postnatal depression was a significant division amongst the women because, for many, pregnancy was a trigger for further problems leading up to candidiasis, which were then compounded by having to look after children rather than concentrate on how to get better. Six out of nine women were diagnosed as having postnatal depression, and three of this group, along with three others, had a history of allergic reactions and ill-health in childhood.

Of the eight women who had not been pregnant, five had a history of a chronic viral infection, sometimes persistent, and only one had had no problems with allergies as a child. The other three had a history of constant childhood health problems which, with hindsight, were clearly to do with allergic reactions to food and weak immunity. Antibiotics were used to treat some of their symptoms, except for three who knew they could not tolerate them. Six out of the nine mothers also had exposure to antibiotics, four over extended periods of time.

Six of the childless group had been put on the pill, ranging from age 14 to 20, in order to regulate periods and minimise extreme pain and discomfort. Gwen, who had had hormonal treatment at 13, was told later that it had stunted her growth, and when she went on the pill in her later teens she had to stop immediately because of weight gain and mood swings. Linda tried the pill twice; each time, after six months she had a migraine which lasted six weeks. Karen developed morning sickness. Veronica started to bleed all the time after a number of years' use. Changing the pill, she put on three-quarters of a stone in weight in three days. Anita was given the pill, age 14, without being told, as part of an experiment; it caused weight gain and thrush.

Although only two in the group of women who had conceived did not experience problems with their periods before getting candidiasis, only one woman was given the pill to alleviate pain. This comparison is not a fair one, however, because for some of the married women the pill was not available when they were in their teens. Two others in this group used the pill as a contraceptive.

On the limited basis of these case studies, it would not be accurate to say that problems were caused by the pill, but it would seem a good idea to design future studies which took account of the role of the pill in making pre-existing problems worse, particularly as it has already been shown that candidiasis affects and is affected by hormonal fluctuations.

An interesting difference between the two groups of women is the amount of tranquilliser use. Six women in the group that had had children were prescribed anti-depressants and tranquillisers, three of whom subsequently had serious problems of addiction and withdrawal. Only two of the childless group were given such medication, one of whom had problems with withdrawal; she had candida with ME.

For Sophie and Jessica, the two women in their 20s who had candida without ME, getting better seemed a 'simple' process of finding the right treatment, i.e. following the anti-candida diet, controlling allergies and, for one of them, taking antifungal drugs.

Jessica's interview is presented in full elsewhere (see pages 19–23). Sophie had a history of asthma as a child, with many antibiotics. A severe attack of glandular fever at 17, lasting a year and also treated with antibiotics, was followed by colitis. Then, four years later, she developed eczema on her hands and face. After trying various elimination diets, she finally consulted Dr Mansfield in 1986, who recommended that she cut out sugar and yeast, and found that she was allergic to house dust. Cutting out sugar brought about a dramatic improvement, reducing her eczema attacks from 75 per cent of the time to one episode a week.

After interviewing the older women, it was not difficult to

imagine that their problems could very easily have been repeated had Sophie and Jessica not found the right diagnosis early on.

12 CASE HISTORIES – OVERLOAD

PAT

Pat's case illustrates clearly the concept of overload; she failed to recover easily from a viral infection, she was exposed to chemical toxicity and, as a result of over-prescribing of antibiotics, she developed candidiasis. The unsympathetic treatment, as she recalls it, from doctors in the early years of her illness would not happen so easily now, but she is left defensively precluded from examining her psychological needs, while her physical symptoms, in need of parallel care, remain undiminished.

I first met Pat in 1986. She insisted on making the journey by public transport to see me, saying that she would be too ashamed to receive me in her own home. Her first gesture was to pull out of her bag a photograph of herself taken on the ski slopes four years before. It was not the same person that sat in front of me. The woman in the picture was slim and alert. The woman I was interviewing was 7 stone heavier and clearly very ill.

The problems seemed to have started when she was 25, working as a laboratory technician for an American company, although four years previously she had had a bad attack of chickenpox which she had taken a year to get over. When she was moved into a small unventilated laboratory she started to feel strangely tired, as if she was losing consciousness. She started to get chest pains, headaches, earaches and sore throats. Her abdomen became bloated, she was constipated and exhausted and she had severe pains in her joints. There was a strange feeling of numbness down her back. At home all she was doing was sleeping. Her doctor prescribed a large amount of antibiotics, after which her weight suddenly and dramatically rose.

Eight months later she had blood and pus in her throat, her pulse rate was 140 and the joint pains were unbearable. Dizziness kept making her fall to the right and her vision was blurring. She had given up going to her NHS GP because he said that viral infections did not last that long, and would only believe that her problems were psychological.

So she consulted a private doctor who had known her for five years, and who happened to have an interest in alternative medicine. He was the first person to express fears about her work environment. At his suggestion Pat asked for a list of all the chemicals in the laboratory. It was refused.

Yet some of her colleagues at work seemed to take her symptoms seriously. Her laboratory manager ordered some blood tests, and it was found that she had raised liver enzymes. Two weeks' sick leave did nothing to relieve the problem. She remembers being too ill to eat.

> I was just lying on the floor. I was living with my boyfriend at that time. He was so distressed I could cry. What he went through. I was out of my brain at this time. I mean, he even thought I was going into a psychotic state because I wasn't coming into a conscious state. And my sleeping pattern was totally different.

Their relationship broke up because of the strain. In desperation one weekend she went to the casualty department of a nearby hospital, hardly able to walk. The doctor she saw said there was nothing wrong with her, although she showed him her abnormal liver results, and he gave her a report saying that she was suffering from liver damage. She collapsed at home and lost consciousness for many hours.

Ten months after her problems started she lost partial vision and was taken to another hospital where she collapsed. She was admitted, and saw three doctors, all of whom gave different diagnoses. Two weeks later she was re-admitted for further tests. The results were abnormal, but the only explanation they could offer was that she was an attention-seeking psychosomatic who also suffered from hysteria. Although her vision returned, she was discharged after a week, still very ill. She had pneumonitis, severe abdominal pain and vaginal bleeding, and she was semi-conscious. A friend accompanying her tried to persuade the doctors that she was unfit for discharge. When they refused to keep her in he took her straight to the Mile End Hospital.

> I remember Rob carried me in, and I remember the casualty sister saying 'You've been very ill, haven't you?' I was treated incredibly. They got a consultant out on call, they did X-rays on call, they did a blood cross-match on call, but luckily I didn't need a transfusion. And they asked me how on earth I could have got myself into that state. They even told me off. I didn't tell them about the other hospital because I thought they might phone up and be told that it was all psychological. They thought it was the IUD.

On the advice of her private doctor she turned down an offer of inpatient psychiatric treatment from the original hospital. He felt that there could be a fungal problem, and she started to take nystatin. The nystatin seemed to be much more effective after she had had six colonic irrigations at a private clinic, although the standard practice of encouraging the good bacterial flora by administering a dose of acidophilus was omitted. Having been tested for allergies, she was found to be extremely allergic to many foods and chemicals, particularly phenol. After seven months she was unable to tolerate nystatin and replaced it with amphotericin.

At this time she was consulting numerous private doctors in a desperate attempt to get to the bottom of her problem. When it was suggested to her by a clinical ecologist that she should leave her job because of her reaction to chemicals, she did not immediately take action.

> Unfortunately I had bought myself a studio flat and was not in a financial position to leave my job. I felt totally trapped. And there was no help on the NHS, only privately. I could not see reason. I felt that I would rather die than be unemployed. So I continued to work to pay for the mortgage. It was my home and if I left I would be homeless. Also I was told that if I was off work again I would not be paid.

But in December, 18 months after the onset of her illness, she was involved in an accident at work caused by her blurred vision. She was reaching up for a bottle of sulphuric acid, knocked over a glass measuring cylinder, and shattered glass entered her eye. She realised that she had to leave her job because if she had dropped the acid she could have blinded herself and others. At the Job Centre, instead of registering her for alternative work, they registered her as disabled and she resigned on medical grounds.

> The financial problems were tremendous. The DHSS would not accept my reason for leaving work or the private doctor's certificate. Soon the bank wanted to repossess my flat – when I stopped work I was £60 short for the mortgage each month, and I already had accumulated debts. The council would not rehouse me. I was in a terrible state. I had no money, soon nowhere to live, no doctor to help me. My GP said that the clinical ecologists were a bunch of con-merchants, and banned me from his surgery. He swore at me actually. He said 'It's totally in your imagination.' The Family Practitioners' Committee said there were no other GPs, and it was my fault for being banned.

Most people by this stage would have given up and returned to their family to be looked after. The problem for Pat is that her sister is a doctor who does not believe in clinical ecology; her father accepts this verdict and accuses Pat of being work-shy, and her mother does not know what to think. Pat is adamant that her family has nothing to offer her. The only contact is an occasional letter from her mother.

Her next move, therefore, advised by the Citizens Advice Bureau, was to initiate court proceedings to sue her former employers and to put in a claim for industrial injury. Both came to nothing. When her lawyers went to inspect her laboratory they found that it was no longer there, and the company failed to cooperate before finally closing down in this country.

The court required her to have an independent psychologist's report and for that she was assessed at St Mary's Hospital in Paddington. To her relief the main conclusion was that her health problems were not psychologically based. Legal aid also paid for her to be tested by Dr Jean Monro; she did a double blind trial with a doctor and a psychologist observing, and it was confirmed that Pat was allergic to many chemicals.

In the end the court agreed that her workplace had caused her illness, but did not agree that the company had been negligent. The industrial tribunal found that her illness was not a recognised industrial disease, and that it could not be an industrial injury because she had not had a specific accident. When she appealed she was not notified of the appeal date, so that she and her solicitor were not able to be present. She lost her case.

Pat made two unsuccessful attempts to retrain, first in law and then in occupational hygiene. She had to give up both courses because she kept collapsing, but the second college did refer her to a consultant in a department of occupational medicine at a leading London hospital. However, when Pat mentioned clinical ecology and allergies the consultant became angry and expressed doubt about the relevance of her exposure to chemicals. Nevertheless he did accept that she was genuinely ill, and diagnosed neuropathy and a vascular dilatory disorder, compounded by depression and frustration as a result of being ill. He declined to treat her, though, because she was already a patient at another hospital. When he wrote to Pat's GP outlining her medical problems as he saw them, the GP's response, while Pat was present, was to screw up the letter and throw it away.

All this time Pat's debts were growing. Her only solution was to sell her flat before it was re-possessed, and find alternative housing in a short-life legalised squat in East London where her condition was not helped by problems of damp and black mould on the walls. In order to get social security she had to pay a clinical ecologist £35 every six months for a medical certificate. This was because the Department of Employment refused to allow her to sign on as being available for work because she had left college because of ill health, and because her NHS GP refused to give her a sick note. There was always the fear that the DHSS would suddenly refuse to accept a medical certificate from a private doctor. Fortunately, when she moved to a new area, she found an NHS GP who was more sympathetic.

Six years after giving up work Pat is still in the same state. She has been receiving sympathetic treatment from the Royal Homoeopathic Hospital, but efforts to help her have failed. Pat commented that she calls her consultant there her 'from-the-waist-up-doctor'; this is because she has been told that she is poisoning herself with her own toxins, but those who treat her seem to ignore her colon. She recalls how much better she felt when she had colonic irrigation, but she has no financial resources to seek such treatment now.

Day-to-day living is not easy:

It consists of struggling to get into a conscious state when trying to wake up. Trying to find the energy to get up, showered and dressed. Exhausted after this, then sitting for hours watching lunchtime TV. Then either back to bed or some shopping. I rarely have the energy to walk to the nearby ones. I catch a bus. I return exhausted, watch TV, then to bed, repeat and so on. Empty, lonely hours stressed with trying to cope financially. Recently I have started two to three hours a week typing training with the local disability centre. Dial-a-Ride gets me there and back.

Pat accepts that the recent publicity about ME may have helped her because she now receives the £20 a week mobility allowance. Although she has been rehoused by the local authority, the quality of her life is immeasurably impaired.

I don't dare explore my feelings on how my life has become, or the future. I have been told I will not recover. My main problem is money. I want to live again – to have a job, money, self-respect and fulfilment. I feel time is running out, my own time-bomb of despair.

I don't think I can allow myself to continue to live much longer like this. It's not that I want to die but that I'm too tired living like this. It's not worth it.

13 CASE HISTORIES – CANDIDA, TRANQUILLISER ADDICTION AND ANTIBIOTICS

Rosemary and Sue experienced the complications of tranquilliser addiction and postnatal depression. Sue's history of repeated antibiotic use was also shared with Rosemary.

SUE

Sue lives in an East Midlands coalmining town, and is in her early 30s. I interviewed her in 1987.

She first got ill when her marriage broke down in 1976; her ear felt frozen, she felt dizzy, sick and shaky. Her doctor said that it was a nervous breakdown and put her on nortriptyline. She had one child at the time. Gradually she got better on her own, and had no problems coming off nortriptyline.

Sue had very painful periods from 11 onwards, requiring time off school and work every month. She also had sinus problems.

> I was always getting a bloated stomach and really bad thrush. I had antibiotic after antibiotic, before and after the tranquillisers. I lived on antibiotics all through those years, to get rid of thrush, catarrh and sinusitis. One kind made me more depressed than the others, which were signs of candida I know now. Some would bring me out in a rash. I'd no sooner have an antibiotic, which would cause the thrush, for which I'd have nystatin, than I'd get nose trouble. So I'd

> have another antibiotic, and so on over the years. I don't touch anything now.

When she met her present husband, in 1980, all her symptoms flared up again but this time they were much worse.

> I went back to the doctor again and came away with Stelazine and another one, which I can't recall. It was an antidepressant. I thought I was depressed when I was told I was depressed; I can always remember, I came away twice as bad as when I went. I told my husband all about it. I took the tablets but I never really picked up, even when I knocked the tablets off.

By the time she wanted another child she had managed to come off the antidepressants by doing it gradually. After the birth she 'started to feel odd' and she was told it was postnatal depression. Coming home with the baby made it worse.

> I brought Charlotte home and after a week I completely went down. I went back to the doctor and he said, 'Oh, it's baby blues.' I got the usual story about 'someone could have a heart attack while I'm listening to you'. My husband is a JCB driver. When I had Charlotte, he was always coming home from work, even though it was difficult. I didn't dare stay on my own because I was frightened I was going to die. I had a thudding in my chest. I was terrified, and I'd be on the phone to him. He'd come, they'd let him, but eventually I realised that I just couldn't keep doing it.

Until six months before the interview she was still on antidepressants, but she felt like a 'zombie' and decided to try coming off them. This time her reactions were stronger, and when she went to the doctor she was told that it was her nerves, and that it would be best to go back on the tablets. She was assured that she wasn't addicted.

> I was addicted. My husband said 'You just can't leave them alone.' My doctor said I wasn't. So it caused an argument between us. Anyway, I went back on them again, taking more and more.

In desperation she went to a naturopath, having seen him advertised in the local newspaper.

> The advertisement was for self-confidence, which I felt I

didn't have. He charged me £10 a time. Funnily enough it did bring some of my confidence out in me. It was like hypnosis. Even though I took these tablets at night, and I felt grotty, I felt as if I was winning. And I told him about the tranquillisers. In the meantime I started getting real bad pains all over me. In fact, it got so bad I could hardly move. I sat down and couldn't get out of the chair. The doctor said that I should have tests at the hospital because I'd got mild arthritis. He gave me arthritis tablets which inflamed my stomach and made it raw. So I had to leave them off as well.

At hospital I had X-rays, and there was nothing at all showing on them to do with any stage of arthritis. When they came back he said 'Yes, you've got arthritis but very mild.' I thought, God, if this is mild what can it be like in 12 months. I couldn't see any future disabled.

The naturopath put her in touch with a local tranquilliser support group. She was advised how to cut down on her pills, and found out that the pain she was experiencing was withdrawal.

The organiser of the group suggested that I was probably suffering from candida and I could get allergy tests. She recommended Dr Kingsley. He confirmed that I'd got candida and that I was also allergic to two or three other things. He gave me a diet sheet. I got back home and I chucked out everything that I shouldn't have.

Her recovery was dramatic to start with; in the first week she lost all her symptoms. This was followed by the disappointment of getting worse, before she started to recover again. On her second visit to Dr Kingsley all that she was left with was pressure in her ears. But further problems arose before her next appointment. 'I had terrible pains, gripping all over me. It frightened me. I was losing a lot of weight.' She could not afford an appointment ahead of time, so she went back to her GP.

He said that it's all right him telling you what to do like this, but all you're getting from him is somebody to talk to. If I was you I'd go away and eat everything you want to eat, and enjoy your Christmas.

By that time I was that down, I did just that. I came home. I started eating what I liked – trifles, cakes, biscuits, chocolates, the lot. Then I was all right over Christmas, until round about the beginning of January. Then all my symptoms started coming back – itching, thrush, everything. I said to my husband, I've just got to go back on the diet, it's as simple as that. I've been on the diet three months now. The only problem is really bad ears and balance. And I'm a little bit itchy. Apart from that I think I'm picking up.

Sue's symptoms are worse in dull, damp and wet weather, particularly her ears. She still gets bad bloating and wind, and occasionally some earaches and nasal congestion. However, she has decided to stop paying for more treatment.

I rely on other people, one or two that I was put in touch with through the support group. We compare symptoms, and different things to try. If it doesn't work we try something else. I've been better on my own, in my own time, in my own way. Some days I know I'm going to have a great day. And other days I get up and I start thinking – this damned diet, when is it ever going to end?

I've got a new GP now. He goes along with me. When I first went on this new diet I told him the diet I was on, and that I intended sticking to it. He gave me some Sudafed for my ear. I took the tablets, and he said if it didn't get better it might need antibiotics. And I told him point blank there was no way that I would take antibiotics. And he questioned me quite thoroughly, and I explained everything to him and he just agreed, and he put it on my card.

Looking back, my candida problems didn't contribute to the break-up of the marriage, but I think I was suffering from candida when the marriage broke up. I was under strain and the candida made it worse. When I look back how I felt at the time, when I was told I was having a nervous breakdown, I think it was the candida. I think that eventually I'd have been well, and just needed a lot of reassurance. I wouldn't have needed any tablets at all.

At one stage before I was diagnosed, my marriage was put through a bad patch. I thought all I wanted to do was opt out, but that passed with perseverance. Because my husband just let it go. I could carry on and on at him, and he didn't bother. He did get mad, but he'd forget.

This was before I was diagnosed. Now I know what I want and I can see the future. I couldn't then. I know what I want

> out of life now, and the things I want to do, and so does he. But before I didn't. I couldn't see any future at all.
>
> I used to feel really ill. When you've got a list of symptoms like that you start to wonder what is happening to you. Most are round the corner now, but I don't worry because I know it's not serious.
>
> Three weeks ago I got myself a part-time job at night sorting out mail for abroad. It's interesting and it makes a change, as well as meeting different people. So I don't feel too bad at all.
>
> I'm plodding along, the same as the others. But I know I'm different because I'm on this diet and they're not. I explained to one, and she just said 'One of them things'. They've all got problems; I thought this diet was a problem till I heard some of theirs.

By 1989 Sue was eating anything she wanted, 'within reason', and was taking regular exercise swimming and dancing. She had changed her job to one with less hours in order to see more of her family. Candida was a thing of the past.

ROSEMARY

Rosemary told me that her health problems started in 1980 when she caught chickenpox. But we quickly went backwards, covering her early life as a young mother and wife, and her struggles to come to terms with her sexual orientation. Although it may seem that stress played a large part in undermining her health, it must also be emphasised that her immunity was damaged by 20 years of tranquilliser addiction.

Rosemary became pregnant at 17 in order to leave home. Her parents refused to let her get married because her boyfriend physically abused her. Within a short time Rosemary met and married someone else, a farm mechanic and manager, who was happy to adopt her daughter. When her first child was two she gave birth to another daughter.

After the birth Rosemary had postnatal depression, for which she was given Valium. She was suicidal and begged to be taken into hospital.

> They put me on Anafranil. I just couldn't cope with these weird thoughts in my head. I found out I was a lesbian. It was very relevant to my life story. The doctor used to push

these feelings aside all the time, and used to tell me that it was my mental attitude, and that it would pass. But it never did. So I lived a lie most of my life.

I'd always known what I was, but I was very naive as a teenager and I wanted to wake up and it wouldn't be there. Because I didn't want to have these strange feelings because I knew my family couldn't cope. I don't care who knows now, because that's me.

I somehow got over this breakdown, but I was never right for years, what with phobias and fears. So anything that went wrong I would just take another pill. I was on Valium for 20 years. The more I took them, the worse they were making me.

After the breakdown she worked in a factory for two years, and then on a smallholding raising chickens. In 1977 she divorced when her children were ten and eight, unable to reconcile marriage with her homosexual feelings. She came to London before this, found a job and began to meet new people, leaving her children in the care of her husband. During divorce proceedings her lesbianism was brought out, as a result of which her family disowned her.

Dave used to bring the children to London to see me but it was very traumatic and heartrending. It used to kill me, to see the children and having to let them go. I didn't want to drag them to London into my new way of life because I didn't think it was fair on them. But also the social worker said that they would be put into a home, or foster parents because of my sexuality. So I didn't have any choice.

Valium was the only way I could cope because I was a really mixed-up woman. I wanted to be heterosexual. With therapy I realised that I had to accept it. I've got a wonderful girlfriend. I'm basically quite happy with my life. I'm independent, I've got a house, a job, a car. Life is now great, but I've just got to get well.

In 1980 I was very, very ill with chickenpox. I'd just got a job in the civil service, and had just given up smoking – I used to smoke quite heavily. I was OK for the first two years after chickenpox, on and off with viruses, nothing too traumatic. But I used to get panic attacks. I didn't know it then, but it was withdrawal from Valium. I saw a programme about tranquilliser withdrawal on television and I

> decided to join a self-help group. I met a few women, and we suffered about two years of withdrawal together.

Then she started getting tonsillitis all the time, having antibiotics every six weeks. This went on for about two years. She was advised by a physiotherapist friend to come off the antibiotics, but because she used to vomit with the tonsillitis she felt antibiotics were necessary. This was accompanied by constant thrush. Having her tonsils out didn't help.

> I was still getting upper respiratory infections, and I started noticing lumps coming up on my breasts. I had to have a lump out. It was benign. This was over a period of four years. I was still taking antibiotics. I was getting off work all the time. In 1986 I had 142 days off. My employers were saying that they didn't know whether they could keep me on.

Hypnotherapy was one of the first therapies that she tried, but it didn't work for her. Then she tried acupuncture for six months, and that helped with her severe headaches. Massage was also helpful at relieving aching muscles. But she felt that she was no nearer understanding the cause of her symptoms.

> I was tested for just about every disease. They even sent me for an AIDS test, which upset me a great deal. My GP did not know what to do with me. She didn't think of the obvious thing that I've got – food. Just talking about it makes me very angry. My friend used to have to come with me. I was in tears because I felt so ill for most days of my life.

More blood tests for glandular fever proved negative. They couldn't locate any virus.

> The symptoms were upper respiratory infections, thrush, tinnitus, sinusitis, I ached all over, my glands were up, exhaustion. I used to sleep for days on end, and I used to get pins and needles, dead legs, jumpy legs. The GP did call it a post-viral syndrome but she wouldn't admit that it was ME.

Rosemary's therapist alerted her to the role of diet, having read an article in the paper about ME. Finally her GP referred her to a consultant microbiologist who specialised in ME. Rosemary had to wait six months, but was eventually told that it sounded like classic ME. Candida was mentioned, but no advice given on how to treat it. Instead Rosemary was told to rest when she needed to and not go into work. Rosemary was indignant:

> Well you can't go through life like that, with three weeks off at a time. I saw the letter she wrote to my GP. She would only recommend that I spend more time and money on luxuries for myself and more time on enjoying life. That was her remedy! I couldn't believe it. To do that more than worrying about going on a specific diet. She didn't think candida was an important part of ME.

Desperate for more advice, her partner paid for her to consult Dr Jenkins at the Royal Homoeopathic Hospital. He said that Rosemary had got candida, and maybe ME as well.

> He found that I've got hypoglycaemia and candida. He said that he wanted me to start on this diet. When I saw it I thought that the world had come to an end. No more this, and no more that. I had severe withdrawal symptoms for a week – I had to have nothing with sugar and yeast in, or any preservatives. I've got it down to a tee now; I can walk past the forbidden foods without being tempted. He told me it wouldn't be an easy process and could take up to three years.
>
> I've been on the diet about 13 weeks. I want to get well and I'm determined to get well. He gave me multivitamins, also magnesium, chromium, evening primrose oil and garlic capsules. I eat garlic every day, and olive oil. For the last two months I haven't had PMT.

Rosemary also changed her GP, having found another practice nearby which was known to be more open, and not prejudiced against lesbians.

> They don't believe in private medicine, so we had a little bit of a hoo-ha – 'I can't take you if you persist in seeing this private doctor.' But after explaining and being in tears, it's helped. But one of the women is still not happy with Dr Jenkins's diagnosis. She's still convinced that I've got ME, and she doesn't really want to know about candida. But the other doctor is more supportive and said that whatever I wanted to do she would support me.

Rest was essential, and Rosemary, with the help of her therapist, decided to put her health first and give up work as an administrative officer dealing with the general public in an employment office. Her partner was prepared to support her until she got better.

> Dr Jenkins wrote my original GP a lovely letter about me and what I've got, but she didn't take any notice. It's a case of having to educate the doctor. I just know that since I've been on the diet I've got up some days and I notice I don't hurt.

Four months after our interview Rosemary rang to tell me that she was consulting a new practitioner, a PhD in behavioural physiology, with qualifications in psychotherapy, Chinese medicine and healing, and with a practice near Harley Street. She had read about him in a magazine, and her impatience to get well overcame her caution about paying more consultation fees. In the first session he took time to tell her about his method of treatment, and to explain that recovery was up to her, with his help. She was greatly helped by his use of colour healing, but her faith in him was shattered when she found out that he was selling Capricin (caprylic acid) to her well above the recommended retail price. She stopped seeing him.

By July 1989 Rosemary reported that she was practically recovered. Although she was still getting throat infections, she was able to throw them off quickly. She didn't need to stick to the diet, although she tried to eat sensibly. The major change had been in her attitude – she talked about the value of being positive and not fighting the illness, but rather going along with it and accepting what your body tells you. Her best move, she felt, was giving her job up. She realised she had had support from her partner, but also felt that it had not all been one sided because she was now able to shop and cook and look after the house. She also had time for her new interests in stamp-collecting and photography.

The change in her psychological attitude to her illness came after she had rested by giving up work, and after she started to feel a bit better than before. She realised that when she stopped seeing Dr Jenkins she was still very impatient. Although she had been disillusioned by her other practitioner, she insisted that he had taught her the valuable lesson that she had to get herself better. 'I know that I had to do it. Other people hadn't said that. You have to listen to your body.'

Rosemary tried to offer help to other ME sufferers by taking them out for a drive or talking to them about her own recovery. She felt depressed by the lack of response that her offers met with, and decided that, rather than expose herself to negative feedback, she would prefer to do voluntary work with the physically handicapped.

The keyword for Rosemary is acceptance, not just in relation to her health, but all areas of her personality and identity. On the other hand, she always believed that change was possible in the end. 'I couldn't sit around and just live with ME. I had to keep trying.'

14
CASE HISTORIES – ONE SYMPTOM AT A TIME

I first interviewed Carol in October 1986. She had an elderly mother to care for as well as her husband and teenage children.

At the time I saw Carol most of the family savings were going on private treatment, after exhausting all the possibilities on the NHS. In 1989, using digestive enzymes, her symptoms had improved so much that she was convinced that an earlier diagnosis of multiple sclerosis was not correct, and refused to accept her GP's view that she was merely in remission.

When Carol was 10 she became ill with rheumatic fever, and spent a year in bed, taking aspirin every four hours, day and night, to lessen the pain. When she started to menstruate it was extremely painful, but she was told it was normal and didn't bother consulting a doctor. Later, when she started work as a nurse, she remembers having bad headaches, and would always have to rest when she got home from work.

Carol's problems really started after pregnancy. She recovered after her son's birth but she didn't 'pick up' after her daughter's. She started to get severe migraines, would cry at anything and had constant colds. This was followed by heart palpitations. Her doctor said that it was just depression after the baby, and gave her the antidepressant amitriptyline. This helped her for some time.

Moving when her daughter was a year old seemed to help both mother and child – the baby had also been ill, with constant tummy bugs and a failure to thrive. But six months after moving, when she had been able to come off her antidepressants, Carol collapsed with a severe pain in her head and lost the sight of one eye for 48 hours.

> I was quite put out by it all and got this strange stiffness in my neck – I couldn't move my neck. So off I trotted to the

doctor again and he said he didn't know what it was really. He thought it was a migraine, and I think from then on I kept getting headaches all the time.

I used to go to bed with a headache and I'd get up with one. I had them continually. Sometimes they were tolerable. I think when you have these things you get so that you live with them. This went on for ages and I got more and more miserable. My father had a brain haemorrhage when he was 50, and I always had this fear at the back of my mind that it could be something to do with that. My doctor said that he didn't think it was very much.

X-rays came back negative, and the specialist diagnosed migraine. Her problems were compounded by continual menstruation, a sore chest and strange pains in her arms. A permanently sore throat went with an intense burning sensation in her mouth and on her tongue – all indications of candidiasis.

Her new GP, unable to connect all the symptoms, sent her to a heart specialist. The day before going she collapsed and she was rushed into intensive care. By this time she had temporarily lost her sight again.

Carol went from one specialist to another, all unable to diagnose what her problem was.

I saw one consultant who turned round and said 'You've got too many symptoms. Just pick one and we'll work on that.' I said to him 'Are you usually rude to people like this?' I felt I must be odd because nobody would believe me, and perhaps it was all in my mind. But when a consultant turns round and says things like that . . . He said nobody could have as many symptoms as that!

Heart specialists couldn't find anything wrong, except that her heart was a bit irregular.

I just wasn't right. I knew I wasn't right. I saw another consultant and he sent me home, saying that he couldn't find anything. I went on for another two weeks and then I collapsed again, and the GP sent me back to intensive care. I stayed there for two weeks while they did all these heart tests.

Then they decided they'd send me to St Thomas's in London for further tests. So I went in this ambulance, with

> a nurse by my side in case I had a heart attack on the way. They thought I had a brain tumour at one time, and I had a brain scan. They couldn't find anything.

Carol usually came back from the tests on a stretcher, because she had passed out. Sometimes her heart rate was up to 140 and she was unable to breathe.

> It was so horrible. I came home and I really couldn't do very much. I couldn't drive the car. And I thought I had had it. I thought I was going to die. I couldn't see any way out of any of it.

Carol's weight dropped to 6 stone from 8 stone, because she was not digesting her food. She had diarrhoea after every meal. The next route was to be tested for lack of stomach acid because they couldn't understand why she had ulcers down her throat.

> But it was the burning in my tongue that I couldn't cope with. I would walk around with a glass of water in my hand because I just couldn't stand it. It was so severe I felt as though I were being choked all the time, as though somebody had their hands round my neck and were strangling me.

Anti-inflammatory drugs helped, and then it was decided that she had an ulcer. After a week or so of taking new drugs they stopped working. Next they thought she had a hiatus hernia. When this proved negative she was sent for further tests in her local hospital. 'They couldn't understand why the drugs weren't being effective. They thought it was because I'd got fed up taking them. They thought I was just queer.'

The ulcers in the throat were examined by an ear, nose and throat consultant. He told her that it was her teeth rubbing her gums, and to go to her dentist.

> He gave me some tablets as he was ushering me out of the door. I was so low and depressed I didn't force him to explain what they were. I just thought, well if he's found out what's wrong with me, and he's got something to cure me, that's fine. It was only after a week of taking them that I found out that they were an anti-depressant. I asked my GP what they were and she told me. In fact they had got rid of the burning, although that was all. I said how can anti-depressants work when that's not really what's wrong with me? 'Oh but it is

> what's wrong with you. When you're depressed you don't recognise that you're depressed.' They filled me up with so much trollop.

Carol continued taking them because they were helping, as well as Ativan to help her sleep, sotalol for her heart, and other drugs for gastric ulcers.

> I just got lower and lower and more depressed. I couldn't sit back on a chair because I hurt. I was so sore in my chest. I had to arrange cushions so that I was in a corner, so my back didn't touch anything. I couldn't lie in bed at night. I used to lie on my side and my husband would prop me up.

Another consultant decided that the throat ulcers were caused by gastric juice, so he advised her not to lie flat. Carol's husband made her some blocks for her to sleep propped upright in bed.

> It was so uncomfortable. This went on . . . it must have been for 18 months. I was so depressed. I cried all the time. I couldn't stand the children. I couldn't pick my daughter up because I hurt so much. I never went out. I took Ativan and amitriptyline for 18 months and you're not supposed to take them for more than three months, and they didn't tell me of any of the side effects.

Although the tests were negative, Carol was told by another specialist that she had multiple sclerosis. He told her that she would be in a wheelchair in two years. Another consultant told her that she had a virus and that it would clear up in time. Looking back, Carol finds it difficult to grasp how a London teaching hospital could not have known about allergies and candida.

The first breakthrough for Carol came when she watched a television documentary, 'Horizon', about allergies in 1985, featuring Dr Jonathan Brostoff from the Middlesex Hospital in London.

> We videoed it and watched it five times. There was so much of me in this programme. My husband said right, stop eating. I was a bit half-hearted about it all, and I didn't see how it could possibly work because it all seemed far-fetched at the time. I didn't think anything would work by that time anyway. I stopped eating and I didn't feel very much better.

Then he said just eat carrots and lamb.

So I lived on carrots and lamb for two days and gradually I began to feel very much better. All the burning went, my neck was better, my joints didn't ache, my arms were better, the angina went, and by the end of the week I was almost fine. Everything had gone except the palpitations, which I couldn't stop.

I didn't know what to do about the drugs, so I kept taking them. This went on for a fortnight and I felt so much better. I didn't dare go to my doctor. She thought I was a nutcase anyway, and this would convince them even more.

I thought there must be something else to this than just allergies. Somebody somewhere must know what this is all about. So I rang the Citizens Advice Bureau and they told me to ring the Green Farm Nutrition Centre. I spoke to Celia Wright, and she said that it sounded as though I had candida. She advised me to see a private doctor who specialised in candida and post-viral fatigue, so I did.

Vitamin and mineral tests found that she was extremely deficient in vitamin B, zinc, magnesium and calcium. She was put on nystatin.

There was very little food that I could tolerate and I couldn't drink anything but water. But I was so much better, and when I started the nystatin the palpitations stopped almost immediately. Gradually I began to feel better.

Carol's attempts to share her new treatment, and her new optimism, with her GP did not go well.

I took all the cytotoxic tests and vitamin and mineral tests to my GP and she laughed and said 'I don't believe in any of this.' I tried to talk to her and tell her what had happened, and how much better I felt, but she didn't want to know. She didn't believe any of it. I wanted a vitamin B12 injection every third day, but she wouldn't give them to me because she didn't believe in it.

I saw Dr Brostoff and he wrote to my GP saying that I needed nystatin, but she wouldn't prescribe it. I tried to tell her how much better I was and she kept looking at me and saying 'You don't look at all well. I think you should go for more tests.' She wanted to prove it was just a remission from the MS that I knew I didn't have. I told her that I was fine.

Having been so ill, it was not surprising that her recovery was not going to be easy. She reacted badly at first to the B12 injections, and food intake was very problematic. She lived on carrots, chicken, lamb, almonds and pears. 'I felt that I would die anyway because of all the reactions I was having to food.'

Taking the nystatin, all the ulcers had gone and all the candida problems. Her periods stopped. She attributed that to her age, 47, but when she stopped the nystatin she started to menstruate again. At our first interview she was still on nystatin after two years, having tried for a month without it when everything started to come back again.

> My palpitations came back immediately, and my ulcers. I was advised to carry on taking it for another two years, but I don't think I'll ever be able to stop it really.

She struggled on her own for a while, unable to pay the medical bills once her doctor moved to London. With partial cover from BUPA, and an arrangement whereby her doctor's partner would sign her BUPA forms because her own doctor was not recognised, she resumed treatment. She was encouraged to have enzyme potentiated desensitisation (see page 165 for explanation of EPD).

At first it seemed that EPD was working. Each time Carol had it she was able to eat anything for about eight weeks. But then she went back to not being able to eat food again. She wanted to understand why and began to feel, in late 1988, that EPD was not tackling the underlying problem. She felt that it was covering up the symptoms and that food was still doing damage. Also, her husband had been made redundant from his job as a lighting engineer and financially it was a difficult time.

> At one stage I just couldn't eat anything and I'd gone lower and lower. All my EPD doctor said was that she expected this with my condition and that she couldn't do anything more for me. She wanted to put me into a private hospital but I had my mother very ill and I just couldn't walk out of my life like that. The feeling was that she couldn't do any more. So I didn't go back.

Carol decided that she would see how long she could go without EPD and nystatin. But she deteriorated, and started to get arthritis very badly.

I just went down and down. Then I put myself on to amino acids. It didn't stop the arthritis but I felt so much better. After that I read Dr Erdmann's book on amino acids, and it seemed so logical and made so much sense.

I went to see him, and had various tests. I was found to be too anabolic, which is linked to osteoarthritis. He gave me sulphur and aloe vera and my arthritis went within four days. When I ran out of the aloe vera my arthritis came back, so I won't stop it again. We couldn't afford to pay for both my daughter and myself, so she had all the tests, and I just had the most important ones. It's helped her enormously. She is 18 and was 6 stone 12 pounds when we started, with continuous diarrhoea. She has a malabsorption problem and, like me, she's not absorbing fats and carbohydrates.

We're both taking digestive enzymes and she started to put on weight straight away and now she can eat everything (we don't eat sugar). She looks well and healthy. He's improved her more than me! I can eat oats now, which is lovely. But I'm not absorbing calcium. All the tests I had showed that I wasn't digesting food properly. I'm sure my father had the same problems. He couldn't put on any weight at all. After a week of being on digestive enzymes for the first time I didn't get headaches after eating.

My stomach acid has completely reversed from being too low to being too high after enzyme treatment. Now the enzymes have been adjusted, and I'm continuing to improve. I still need to rotate my food all the time. Since installing filtered water I no longer need to urinate every hour and my sleep is much improved.

It's too early to say what the outcome will be, but everyone else I've seen treats allergies, whereas my impression is that Dr Erdmann treats what causes the allergies. Clearly, candida was only part of my problem, but my doctor still doesn't recognise it, even though I'm so much better.

15 CASE HISTORIES – TURNING POINTS

Anita and Erica have a history of problems going back to childhood, making it very difficult for them to conceive of living without having to be aware of their bodies and the restraints put upon them by ill health. In trying to get better they didn't know what to aim for, simply because they didn't know what it was like to be healthy.

Anita tackled her problems on all fronts, after first experiencing some relief from candidiasis when taking caprylic acid. Erica, after reaching a point of desperation and despair, turned her health around by strengthening her religious faith, and realising that change was possible if she applied herself to finding answers; waiting for others to give her the solution would not necessarily happen. Each woman had a different life-situation which affected the course of the illness and the types of problems that they faced. Anita was living alone and struggling to support herself; Erica was supported within a caring relationship, but at the same time was struggling to care for her children, despite her unreliable health.

ANITA

At the time of the first interview in 1987 Anita was 42. Throughout our subsequent meetings she was living on her own, with a brief interlude when she started a relationship. Her work had always been in the caring professions or the media but, because of health problems, from 1980 onwards she was unable to keep a job for long. When I first met her she was working for a housing charity for the institutionalised, but her low tolerance for stress and her increasing ill health made her give up work. In 1989 she felt well enough to go back to work, this time to a more manageable job in a library. Her choice of jobs was restricted because of her extreme reaction to cigarette smoke.

Anita was not breastfed as a baby. She was a fussy eater as a child and allergic reactions may account for her extreme fatigue.

> I remember waking up as a child and my whole body would be throbbing and I would be absolutely exhausted. I couldn't get up. And Father used to get so angry with me, and say that I was lazy, trying to avoid school. He didn't have any understanding at all. That still happens. All through my life, throbbing and exhaustion as though I'd run 20 miles in the night.

She feels that difficulties in her relationship with her father could have stemmed specifically from the fact that she was always ill as a child, but without being believed.

> I was always accused of exaggerating to get attention. He forgets that I had very severe ear problems from the age of two to twelve. He thought I was over-dramatic. I used to make him search the house for smells of gas. I used to smell fungus. I used to drive him up the wall.
>
> My father was a very healthy person and he just didn't have room for any other sick person in the family, apart from my mother. He would accuse me of putting my thermometer in the tea and stuff like this. No wonder I had a bad relationship with him. So the stress was always constant, you couldn't get away from it.

She was prescribed numerous courses of antibiotics for her ear infections. She remembers screaming in agony, and banging her head against the cot. They lasted until she was 12, and as a result she has had bad scarring of the eardrums. Her schooling was affected.

> I remember trudging up to the hospital. I had to go twice a day. They used long pieces of gauze dipped in gentian violet, and they used to stick them down my ears with enormous great forceps, masses and masses and masses of it every day. It cut into my schooling and everything. It seemed to last for an eternity. I have a very very bad memory of a lot of this. Bits come back to me. I think I've learnt to block it out. I remember hardly any of my childhood and I think it was mostly because it was incredibly painful.

Anita's periods were normal for the first year, after which she had many problems. She saw a gynaecologist when she was 14, who put her on the pill without disclosing what it was – she was just given a 'daily pill'.

> Later he told me and I was so cross. I was absolutely furious. On the pill my period pain stopped. I got a period for two days, but it was like chocolate glue and it itched like mad. I can only imagine that that was thrush.
>
> They took me off the pill because it had been an experiment, and there was nothing else to give me. So I was dismissed. Without the pill the period pain was so bad I used to go to bed for more than two days. Agony. My mother understood what I was going through. My father didn't. Eventually I did go back on the pill, willingly. I got to the stage where the pain was paralysing, so I took it to take the pain away, which it did. But it made me fat and depressed, and lots of other things. Thrush certainly got worse.

Eventually she was told by a professor that she had to stop taking the pill because the hormones were affecting her badly and she was getting very high blood pressure.

Various specialists tested various parts of her body, all finding nothing wrong. Visits to gynaecologists were particularly frequent. As she got older she found she had more and more strange reactions to foods, pollens and mould.

> I worked at Capital Radio and couldn't drink their coffee. My whole mouth came up in ulcers. I don't know why. I couldn't connect anything with anything. In an advertising agency job my arms were aching like mad for no apparent reason. Something happens to me in the spring; I wake up with aches in the spine. In September I have to keep away from the harvest.

After an injury to her hip Anita started having continuous problems in her joints and spine. She was eventually seen by a rheumatologist, who said that she didn't have arthritis.

Food reactions were particularly severe. If anything disagreed with her, her saliva glands reacted immediately, and she felt sharp shooting pains in her mouth so that she had to spit the food out. Fresh garlic and vitamin C helped enormously, but not enough to prevent bad flatulence with all foods, sometimes resulting in agony well into the early hours of the morning. It meant that she gave up eating socially, unless she took her own food. And other areas of her life were also affected.

> My hobby is/was sculpture and pottery, but I haven't done any for ages. I stopped sculpture. I'd be banging away and when I stopped I found that I couldn't open my hand to release the chisel or the mallet. I had to ease my fingers open and spend ages getting life back into my arms. Everything was stiff. The same thing happened after a short time holding the phone. I had to stop pottery because the clay started to affect me. I don't have any hobbies any more. I really miss sculpture very badly.
>
> Going out in the evenings, I can't tolerate any smoke; I go into a total spasm. Bright lights affect me very badly too. My eyes get very sore. I'm hypersensitive to noise. In the cinema I can't hear 50 per cent of it because of the echo. I gave that up a long time ago because of that problem. I have almost permanent tinnitus. My enjoyment now is going to see my friends, or them coming to see me. But there are definite rules – I had to give up alcohol. I really am very limited in what I can do. I very rarely go out in the evenings. I come home at seven or eight. I'm really worn out. I can't do anything. I can't walk around much.

In the first interview I asked Anita if she felt that food was dominant in her life.

> I feel that it is my life. I always have the feeling that there is something ruling me, even as a kid, though I didn't know what it was. I used to think it was my periods.
>
> Sometimes I have a sense of humour, and other times when I talk to people they get this overwhelming sense of grief when they meet me because my sense of it is so overpowering.
>
> That's something that I became very aware of at one stage and it's made me withdraw a lot. So it's a big, big, big problem and I don't know where it goes from here.
>
> I used to be very committed to things. I've opted out of everything now. I don't volunteer to do anything.

When Anita was 40 she was sterilised voluntarily. During the operation her Fallopian tubes were removed altogether because they were infected. The cause of the infection was not established, but Anita's feeling is that candidiasis played a role. Her view is strengthened by the fact that after the operation her symptoms of food and chemical intolerance, muscle fatigue and exhaustion increased. She also had menopausal symptoms of hot sweats.

> This recent onslaught, it's now been constant, it has a life of its own. It's getting bigger. It's not going away. It's getting worse. The sterilisation is the only factor that I can pin down that could explain it.

The first indication that she might have allergies came when she saw a TV programme which featured Dr Jonathan Brostoff of the Middlesex Hospital in 1985.

> I had so many emotions, every emotion that I've ever experienced. It was incredible. Suddenly there was someone who knew what had been happening to me for years and years. I was on the phone to the Middlesex the next day. I was determined that I was going to track something down. By my own means I got an appointment with Dr Wraith at St Thomas's Hospital, who had a much shorter waiting list than Dr Brostoff. At the same time I also decided to try an alternative treatment, so I went to the British College of Naturopathy and Osteopathy.

The BCNO gave her a diagnosis of candida in three visits over a period of three weeks. Doctor Wraith at St Thomas's made the same diagnosis in the same number of visits, but each visit was three months apart; this was because he only worked at the hospital half a day a week, unpaid. The NHS gave him an office, allowed him to use a staff nurse, a sister and two receptionists, and that was all. His first diagnosis had been that she suffered from multiple allergies, and then he came to the view that candida involvement lay underneath. This was reinforced by the fact that she reacted badly to Marmite and cheese, and had persistent vaginitis.

Anita started on a diet which seemed to work. She made charts of food intake and immersed herself in reading about clinical ecology. Her doctor suggested that she take nystatin, explaining what it was. Anita did not like the idea, but she eventually went on it in November 1986, because of her bad reactions on holiday during harvest time. At the time of our first interview she was still taking nystatin, with very bad reactions. Her doctor encouraged her to persist with small amounts, but in the end she stopped after six months.

> I read reports in the National Research into Allergy newsletter of people praising nystatin like mad. All I know is, when I started it, it made me a lot worse. Whether I'm allergic to nystatin or whether it's the toxins which are being released in the body, I don't know, but it felt as though I was being poisoned. I felt that I'd been taken over. I now call the yeast my little extra-terrestrial, my universe invaded.

Anita had tried to talk to her GPs about candida, and was grateful when they listened.

> They say where is it. And I try to explain what candida does in the body. The woman doctor tries not to be condescending about it. But the man is just unbelievably so. You have a seven-day course of nystatin to get rid of candida and that's it, and then it's gone, and you either have it in your mouth or in your digestive tract or vagina.
>
> My GP knows it exists, but she believes it's thrush. I think she's somebody who, if it could be described scientifically and in less emotional terms – because when I see her I'm very uptight – I think she would be prepared to sit down and listen. The other GP, who is male, wouldn't.
>
> The first sign of thrush I go to my GP for the bits and pieces. Whenever I get flu I go and see her because I told her that I wanted a record of whenever I was unwell. I felt that there was something wrong with my immune system, and it had been like that all my life. She thought this was a bit boring first of all, and then she realised – I kept turning up in a terrible state – that I was getting all these colds and flus and things. Now she hasn't seen me for a while. She's going to put it all down to the fact that I've got a job, and that my problems were psychosomatic. I know she is. She's not hoity toity with it. She's very sweet and nice, so I'm lucky.

In her second interview, six months after the first, Anita was beginning to feel that there may be a link between her allergies and emotional states.

One-and-a-half years later we met for our last interview. In the intervening period Anita had managed to make several positive interventions in the course of her illness. Despite the fact that she was unemployed and very short of money, she had managed to find alternative therapists who would help her for reduced fees.

The first change that was significant was taking caprylic acid (Capricin was not easily available at the time). It was not recommended by any doctor or therapist; she found out about it when reading the Candida Albicans Advice Group newsletter.

> I started to feel a lot better. Then I had the energy to go for things like reflexology, hypnotherapy and spiritual healing. I had to have something to bring me to that level. For me caprylic acid was the most important thing. The other things came after that.
>
> Hypnotherapy helped sufficiently for me to be able to see beyond my family situation and to feel a bit easier about things. Mostly it's to do with conflict, and perpetually being made to feel that there really was nothing wrong with me even though I felt that there was something wrong with me. Being at loggerheads. It wasn't that I wanted attention as a child. I got masses and masses of attention. It was there all the time, you couldn't escape from it. I can now recognise that it wasn't that, and I no longer have to try and prove it to other people because I can see it myself. I think I used not to be able to see that.
>
> I was going to see someone for kinesiology, but I didn't pursue it because at the first interview she explained that she would teach me to do things for myself, and at that time there was no way that I could do anything for myself because my memory was so appalling. And also my will. I had just enough to get me there but not enough to do what she wanted.

Although Anita was on a low income she was saving money because she was too ill to go out. However, she was spending a great deal on supplements. Her mother used to help out and, since going back to work, Anita has been able to pay her back.

Anita managed to get her GP to refer her to the Royal Homoeopathic Hospital. Her doctor offered her enzyme potentiated desensitisation, but only on condition that she take nystatin first. Anita managed to avoid doing so, and was subsequently started on EPD. Because she was already starting to feel better she finds it difficult to assess what effect EPD had. She had injections every three months, and each time she suffered extreme reactions. Now the intervals between are extending and she is sure that it helps.

Spiritual healing was also of benefit, particularly during a setback brought on by deciding to eat anything.

> I think what happened was that the Christmas before last I decided that I was going kill or cure, and I started eating absolutely anything I wanted, and it nearly killed me. I got pneumonia, and they diagnosed that I was also asthmatic. I realised that I'd completely overdone it and I had to slow down.
>
> I have to admit that at that time I did have suicidal thoughts. I was getting fed up with the whole thing, fed up with the fact that I couldn't go anywhere, that my life had virtually come to a standstill. My friends had virtually left me. I'd had to give up work. My family got very fed up, to a point where my younger sister repeatedly called me a parasite. My older sister was very supportive.

Other sources of support seemed to be absent. Her consultant at St Thomas's retired, without a replacement. Her GP didn't seem to understand, and the Candida Albicans Advice Group was not able to respond to telephone calls when she needed advice. She hadn't yet started at the Royal Homoeopathic Hospital. One particular healer helped her enormously, encouraging her to carry on when her fear was that she would give up again.

Coming through the crisis was helped by a breakthrough in her relationship with her father.

> The watershed was when I blurted loads of things out, about my childhood. This was after going to the hypnotherapist. My father said something nasty to me and I just dissolved into tears. I used to be stiff upper lip, and stand there and take it.
>
> I've had psychoanalysis and psychotherapy, but I didn't get much from them. I would try to confront my father but I never found the right way of doing it. Eventually I found a way of doing it by accident, which was to burst into tears and be vulnerable. And he then became totally vulnerable. It just happened. I felt terribly sad at the end of it because

I told him that I could never remember him telling me he loved me. I could never remember him telling me he was proud of me, and I could never remember him cuddling me.

He was sitting next to me, and I was sobbing. It reminded me that when I was a child I sobbed uncontrollably. I used to cry desperately, with my parents and on my own.

Eventually my mother said to my father, aren't you going to say something to her, and he looked at her like a big idiot, as if to say what do you mean? She motioned to touch me, and he very tentatively put his hand on me. It was as if he was either touching something that was going to break, or he was approaching something that was going to give him an enormous rejection. And he put his fingers, not his hand, on my shoulder. I realised that that was as much as I was going to get, so I responded and put my arm right around him.

I think he had been frightened of me. I felt very sorry for him because I realised that he couldn't tell me that he loved me and he couldn't tell me that he was proud of me. What he did say was that he had been proud of me while I was fighting for my health. And that was the first indication that he recognised that there was anything wrong with me. I thought fair enough. There was no reason for me to ask him to give his all. But I felt much better afterwards. I felt it was terribly sad that we had grown so far apart and he still couldn't say it.

But he does still need to be reminded not to smoke in front of me, and to do the washing when I am away. [Anita reacts to some washing powders.] He'll say yes now, rather than this is a load of rubbish. I think he thinks I'm still bonkers.

I think I've discovered that I'll do anything I can to run away from conflict. Which I now think is why I've never been able to sustain relationships. Because the family conflict was so much on top of what was already going on on the sidelines. It's only now at the ripe old age of 44 that I am beginning to see these things.

Now I can see that I used to recreate the stress in all situations because I wanted to see if I could break the pattern and escape from it. Within the relationships that could break the pattern, and allow me to escape from it, I would carry on and see them as friends. And those that perpetuated it in the same way as the family did I would escape from.

Now that I've removed a variety of things from my life, I'm beginning to see more clearly. And becoming more aware of the things that I need. I'm becoming much more aware of the fact that I do need a relationship. But I'm not going to do anything that is going to throw me into one. There's no way that I'm going to become desperate about it. Then I would stand a chance of repeating something. I've always avoided relationships. I have them, but when conflict arose I would want to run away.

I can only see that now. There are loads of things that I couldn't see before. I would never have admitted before that I was an addict to sugar. Coming off it is going to be as hard as it was coming off cigarettes, if not worse. But it's only me that can stop it. I was eating it on and off in patches throughout the illness.

Anita now works in a children's library. It allows her creative skills to be used because she can make things. Her position is threatened by financial cutbacks, but she is determined not to go back to unemployment. Her strategies for coping take account of her remaining limitations.

First of all it was tiring. So I asked to save the sitting down jobs for the evening. That way I managed to crawl through. Now it's a different tiredness, an expected tiredness, whereas before it was exhaustion, and doubt about whether I could get home.

I need to keep away from allergens, and from stress. Being a library assistant meets those conditions. That will play a big part in allowing me to slow down. I've discovered that my pace is very very slow. Whereas before I would rush round half doing things and then getting too tired, I now realise that if I move very slowly and horribly methodically I get through what I need to get through. It's important to find techniques to allow me to control the situation rather than the other way round. That's one of the big secrets.

Now that I've taken myself away from this compulsive instinct to work in the caring professions, things are better. I really have felt that I've needed to care for other people and in doing so I have continued to make myself ill, because I've been taking on too much. I was trying to say to myself, you need to be cared for. Not that you need people to be sorry for you, or to fawn over you, or to rush around and say please

> let me do everything for you, but for people to understand and care about the fact that I really was feeling dreadful, even though I couldn't perhaps explain it or show it.
>
> That's maybe why I went into psychiatry because that was the nearest point to that area. I was a nursing assistant in the psychiatric day hospital for a year and a half. I adored it there but I had to leave because the salary was so awful.
>
> The fact that I would like to train to be a healer is aiming in the old direction, but if there is something in my personality that needs to care for people maybe that's a good way to do it because the boundaries are very strict.

Contemplating her candida she had the following to say:

> It's still there, but well under control. But I've not seen the last of it. At least it is under control. I understand about it now. I'm not flapping about in the dark any more. When people say to me now they think it's all psychosomatic I think to myself, OK, psychosomatic is body and mind and the two work together, and I see it in a totally different way to the way they mean it.
>
> So I've learnt a lot that's helped me to cope with it in a far far more objective fashion. That, I think, is half the battle, because nobody else is going to tell you what's going on, unless you happen to fall in the hands of the right person. That's probably the biggest confusion. How to start, where to start. If I wanted to be 100 per cent well I'd still be on that wretched diet that I was on. But there has to be a quality of life. I'm feeling so much better than I was, I don't mind if I lapse as long as it's above a certain level.
>
> Dealing with the emotional aspects has allowed me to get rid of the tension inside, at the same time as getting treatment for the candidiasis. They've all been pegging upwards, some alternately and some together. I think if I hadn't tried to do the two things, I would still be down there somewhere because I think the two things are linked. It would be impossible to say that there's no connection. I'm not totally there. If I can maintain where I am now I shall be happy. If I can get better I shall be happier still.

ERICA

Erica is 54, and married with three grown-up children. She

lives in a south-east seaside town, and she runs a nutritional consultancy from home. This work grew out of her own experience with candida and ME.

Reading her case history it is impossible to ignore the relevance of her Christian beliefs. Her views are deeply held, and I was impressed by the positive part that her conviction played in her decision to turn around her past history of health problems. Her experience has left her determined to help others.

As a child Erica was always away from school with constant colds and bilious attacks. She was an only child and her mother was sympathetic to her health problems, partly because she shared some of them herself. She became school phobic because of her terror of doing gymnastics. (Her problems with balance she now ascribes to candida.) As a teenager she hated being away from home, and completely lacked self-confidence.

In her teens her constant colds turned into permanent sinusitis, and a fall on stone steps was the start of 30 years of back problems. 'It was just something else I couldn't rely on.' Her back problem has now cleared, and she feels that this is because her injury was colonised by candida, which she has now eliminated with appropriate treatment.

After she married, more and more symptoms developed, including devastating allergies. Her description of her symptoms sounds remarkably like ME.

> I was ill for a whole year in 1969, just after my third child. If I went to the shops on the corner I would have to spend the rest of the day in bed. At the same time I was trying to cope with the family. Doctors didn't come up with anything. The other children were seven and five. It was quite tough. As soon as the baby was born I developed gallstones. It took the doctors six months to agree that it was anything other than postnatal depression, so I lived with terrible pain. After six months I had private tests and it was diagnosed.

At the same time the baby developed pyloric stenosis, only diagnosed after five weeks.

After the year of overriding weakness she discovered that she was allergic to North Sea gas, whose installation coincided with her fatigue. At that time all the doctors pooh-poohed the idea.

I knew it was gas because I kept out of the kitchen for a week and got better. We took all the gas out of the house and I got better, till I went where there was gas, in houses and shops. Often I wouldn't know it was there. I would be out for the count for about five days, and when this happened it was usually because I had been unknowingly in contact with gas.

By 1972, although we had got rid of the gas, many other allergies had developed and I was in a terrible state, both physically and mentally. I was in a constant anxiety state because, although I was a Christian, I didn't know whether God ever meant me to be well.

I'd always fought against my ill health. Most candida and ME people are fighters. To achieve anything at all they have to be. I was teaching Sunday school, doing women's meetings, and from time to time working. But it was a constant struggle. I had a very, very supportive husband and parents. But I was getting constant sinusitis, constant fibrositis, constant tummy upsets, vaginitis, and flu attacks and allergic reactions all the time.

From March to July every year I would feel really ill, including a feeling of heaviness and uselessness which attacked all my limbs. The first time this happened I was rushed to the National Hospital for Nervous Diseases for tests, but nothing was discovered. After a few months the symptoms went, only to return the next year, so we began to realise that allergy was involved. In addition to all this there were many teeth problems and constant back problems. There was never a day without one or more symptoms to cope with.

Somehow we did cope. But I could never rely on being able to collect the children from school. You get a very funny psychological self-image. You feel ashamed of yourself. People say I won't ask you how you are because you're always ill. These things go deep. And you just think that's how I am. But no one had any idea of the fight it was just to keep going, to try and live a normal life.

In 1972 I hit rock bottom, physically and mentally. It just struck me one morning in church – I was shaking uncontrollably with an anxiety state – that this was ridiculous. As a Christian, if I really believed the Christian message, I ought to be experiencing joy, peace and victory in life. I knew I'd got to sort things out at that level. I had got to apply myself to seeking answers. I prayed as never before. I came to realise that it wasn't God's purpose for me to be as I was. His purpose was for me to be in victory over the situation.

That was the beginning of my uphill climb and I began to get on top of the anxiety state. Now there was hope. That psychological breakthrough was the first important thing that happened.

I received the laying-on of hands for healing from a Christian minister. I felt tremendous peace, and when he went I looked down at my Bible and it said 'God will keep all sickness far from you . . . Little by little you will overcome your enemies.' I just knew that was God's promise for me. I've hung on to it through thick and thin. If I come over with a positive attitude it's because of that. It's so real to me. Whatever bad times that I've had to go through since then, I've hung on to the promise from God and it has made all the difference. I had a certainty that one day I would be completely well, and that's what has brought me to where I am now.

I was completely healed of my gas allergy. I came off the antihistamines and suffered terrible reactions but I've never had a gas reaction since then. We've even reinstalled gas heating now. What threw me at first was why I should be healed of that, and not the other problems, for it soon became clear that they were still around!

Linking nutrition with health was a revelation which came when a friend lent her a book by Adelle Davis, *Let's Cook It Right* (Unwin, 1963).

Up to then I honestly hadn't thought about what I was feeding myself or my family. Through Adelle Davis I learnt about low blood sugar (I certainly had that) and how to control it by diet. And I learned how to control allergic reactions with vitamin supplements. It was a real breakthrough and things began to improve. But there was still a long way to go.

Then she read about yeast, and suspected that that might be a cause of some of her problems. 'I knew it had been there all my life because my earliest memory, aged three, was of being sat in a bowl of something because I was sore.' Her doctor did not agree and would not prescribe nystatin.

> He said he would give me some vaginal cream (again!) and if it didn't clear up in a week it couldn't be thrush. I said that I'd been doing a lot of reading about it, and he said you don't get knowledge from books, you get it from experience. When the condition didn't clear he sent me to a gynaecologist, because the problem was 'obviously to do with my age'.

The gynaecologist agreed that Erica probably did have a candida infection and carried out an operation to cauterise her cervix, which made no difference. Erica's next step was to do something for herself, because of her GP's attitude, and she followed an anti-candida diet. Although she was sure this was the right thing to do, it did not make any difference. Then two years later she transferred to another GP who was interested in candida.

> I was on nystatin for a year and a half, with an even stricter diet. For a couple of months I experienced a great deal of die-off, but overall it didn't make much difference. I still had extremely low resistance to infection and constant vaginitis. The Christmas before last I had a virus and I was still ill with it in April.

Reading a back copy of *Here's Health* she found out about a research project in which volunteers were needed to try Capricin (caprylic acid) to treat candidiasis. Her local chemist found the supplier, she sent for information and, on that basis, put together a programme of Capricin, bifidobacteria and diet.

> At that time it was thought you had to be on maximum dose, and the die-off symptoms I experienced for the first two months were horrific – physically and mentally. Now you are recommended to start on a low dose and build up. But I stayed with it. Suddenly after two months, I found stamina that I had never had in my life before.

This coincided with her husband going away for three months on a residential training course.

> I was still a very dependent person because of my ill health. Letting my husband go on the course was the hardest decision I've ever had to make but I knew it was what God wanted. I had to be dependent on God instead of my husband. It was incredible, because from the day he went things really started to get better. People who saw the change in my

health started to ask me for advice. My doctor was delighted, and arranged for me to be the agent for Lamberts and BioCare. I started placing orders and supplying people and generally finding myself in a consultancy situation. I grew busier each day and had the strength to do it all! I didn't have time to miss my husband!

I couldn't supply Capricin without explaining to people what it was all about. So I registered to start the Institute of Optimum Nutrition course. It is very demanding. Then a local paper did an article about ME, and I wrote in to talk of my experience, with the result that they did an article on me. I had 70 replies because the epidemic is so rife. Some didn't want to know when they saw the diet sheet.

Erica stayed on Capricin for six months because she still had some minor symptoms, even though she felt so much stronger. She began to introduce foods such as bread and cheese, without the previous allergic reactions. Taking butyric acid complex also helped. After several months of relaxing her diet some of her symptoms returned and she went back on Capricin.

For a couple of years I had a really painful elbow. After two months on Capricin it went. Now, since I've gone on Capricin again I've had an outbreak of ringworm, as though it's been pushed out to the surface. It just shows why you need to be ongoingly sensible with the diet, because if yeast is hidden in joints it's going to take quite a while for it to come to the surface.

I have recently tried a new product called Catalase Enzyme Complex to help with my allergic symptoms, and it has made a tremendous difference, although it is too soon to tell permanently. Oxy-Pro has also helped – it is designed to be absorbed under the tongue, in order to reach yeast problems in the head more directly than Capricin. It's working to clear my mouth and sinuses of yeast once and for all.

I have discovered that a lot of people with ME are really very much like me, with unreliable health and chronic fatigue, and 'flu' several times a year lasting for long periods at a time.

The reason I was in a bad psychological state was because anxiety got hold of me because I didn't know whether I was ever going to get better. But after my crisis I had a certainty about that. It has taken a long time – from 1972 – and I've been through a lot of bad health in the mean time. It would have been very easy sometimes to have given up, yet somehow I knew I never could. I was obviously meant to wait for the Capricin and the other new products coming out of ongoing research.

Here am I, a grandmother, running a consultancy, a business, and studying for a diploma. It's unbelievable when you think how I was till just over a year ago. I used to be a secretary and PA but I usually had to leave each job because of health problems. Now I've got all these people dependent on me, and it doesn't frighten me in the least because my health is now reliable, and I know I can depend on God.

16
CASE HISTORIES – MOVING ON

Juliet and Gwen are free of symptoms and describe themselves as better. What worked for them is not necessarily the right formula for others, but their willingness to try various options with an open mind helped them to discover how to get help from others while helping themselves.

JULIET

I heard of Juliet through a friend, and was curious to interview her because of her positive experience with a healer. She has one son who is in his 20s and a 14-year-old daughter. Before Juliet became a healer herself, she was an actress and a sculptor.

Juliet began having rashes on her neck in 1986, spreading to her legs and then all over her body.

> My feet itched, and there was terrible itching up the bowels. The doctor thought it was worms. He gave me sleeping pills, because he said if I slept I couldn't itch.
>
> On holiday in Italy I was very ill, and in hospital I was given very strong cortisone pills, which helped. When I came back the doctor said that it was not terminal and that it would go. He didn't seem interested in treating me at all.
>
> My husband got very cross and sent the GP a complaining letter, because we had been with them for ages. They referred me to St Thomas's Hospital. I saw a terribly nice man but he didn't believe that there was anything wrong with me.

In desperation Juliet went to a private allergy clinic and had tests. They showed that she was allergic to everything except honey. Dr Jean Monro diagnosed candida, but the treatment had little effect, except for nystatin. The rash always came out at night, and was made worse by stress. Juliet had to give herself injections, which Dr Monro called cocktails, of all the things that she was allergic to. They didn't help.

I was put on a rotation diet. I liked that, though I lost a tremendous amount of weight and that was dreadful. It wasn't helping at all. I got terribly thin.

Then someone told me about a healer called Lily Cornford. So I thought, if I go, nobody need know. It won't interfere with all these people who aren't interested.

It was fantastic. Healing brought out the rash, made it much much worse. It was like the poison being drawn out of my body. After the initial thing of getting much worse, it got better. After three months the rash was completely gone. Getting worse is sometimes a natural process, I've learnt.

I'm absolutely amazed that I wasn't given tranquillisers in the state I was in before the healing. I used to be on them years ago a lot. The doctors knew I was that sort of person. A lot of them thought it was the change of life.

I was in a depressed state when I was ill. You're tired, you're depressed, and feel awful. After I went to the healer I didn't have to keep to a special diet. I could eat anything. It was the same with the nystatin. When I started with the healer I stopped taking it.

I was a bit frightened of going to be healed because I didn't know anything about it. There was a little elderly white-haired lady in Kilburn who talked to me. I discovered later that they heal through colour. Certain colours represent cleansing colours; for example spring green or sapphire blue. Calming colours. You think of these while focusing on different energy points of the body. It really works.

It was a tremendous feeling of love, extraordinary – most of it was through a love energy. Getting in touch. A lot of it is counselling. After I was better I realised that it was absolutely fantastic, that I'd been helped so tremendously. I wanted to help other people, so I trained to be a healer and now I'm working with Lily.

I think we all have the ability to heal. It's part of the process of life. I haven't got healing hands particularly. I'm just being an instrument. I'm receptive to it, and it comes through. If we think of the right things it comes through.

When I went to Lily's I said I know it's my responsibility, I'm ill because I've made myself ill. She said getting better needs to be 70 per cent yourself and 30 per cent someone else helping you. I think you have to take the responsibility yourself. But some people find it terribly hard. When you're not depressed it's easy to think of something lovely. When you are depressed, you can't get that cloud away from you. And that's when you need help. Pills don't help because they stop the flow of the mind and the body. That's why healing helps because it unblocks and allows the joy to seep through, and that takes the cloud away.

I'd always suffered from allergies of some sort. Allergies are to do with your space being invaded, which is the same as candida. You don't have your centre. Most of us don't make time for ourselves. You have to love yourself to make yourself well in order to be able to help other people, or give.

I've always worked with my hands, dressmaking, sculpting, acting with my body. I was out of work for a long time but you have to go through bad patches to learn. That's the purpose of being on the earth, to learn from bad things. I'm so grateful that I had candida. Without that I wouldn't now be healing. It's completely changed my life. If I hadn't been ill that wouldn't have happened. I think that's wonderful. It forces us to recognise things that we take for granted.

I consciously know why I got ill, but don't consciously know why I got the feeling that it was my responsibility to get well. That's what I find the hardest feeling to give people whom we treat. I suppose I had a difficult time with doctors, and the allergy treatment, and the professor at St Thomas's who thought I was making it all up. They must have given me this 'me' thought. Because no one else had managed to help me. Therefore it's very good that they'd been so negative because if they'd been positive . . . maybe I had to go through that process.

GWEN

Gwen is French but has lived in England since her early 20s. She is 37 and was first interviewed in 1986. She gave up teaching in 1988 in order to train to be a Gerda Boyesen therapist. In 1985 she won the Action Against Allergy essay competition, and excerpts are reproduced here.

She had been alerted to the need to sort out her problems with food after a serious car accident when she had fallen asleep at the wheel after eating Kendal mint cake (pure sugar). Coffee gave her headaches, her usual school lunch of a cheese sandwich gave her muscle tremors around the eyes, blocked sinuses and 'brain fag', and she was no longer able to tolerate any alcohol. She consulted Patrick Holford at the Institute of Optimum Nutrition but elimination diets did not help.

Recognising that her allergies and inability to cope may be to do with stress, she gave up fulltime teaching to concentrate on her MA studies and her health. Inadvertently she walked past an AAA symposium on candida and sat down to participate.

> 'You have to be your own detective' Dr Crook had urged us during his talk on recent studies of causes and effects which could be attributed to candida yeast. Out of his list of ten I had then scored a potential seven; so had most women present at the symposium. True, I had had colitis, was suffering from chronic constipation, had always had irregular periods and could not bear the pill – but I had never taken antibiotics. True, I also had low thresholds of tolerance, and generally lacked stamina, feeling dozy after meals. Like my mother, I was also a born pessimist – and a sceptic.
>
> Lacking conviction (and proof), as with any wild story one hears for the first time, I had shelved my notes soon after. It was not until I developed athlete's foot for the second time in 12 months that, puzzled, I went to take another look at them. Weren't those American researchers simply being enthusiastic in their willingness to explain away some commonplace troubles? I bought the cheapest of the available books on the subject and found out that I had been overlooking one of the most embarrassing but telltale symptoms – rectal itching, preceded in my case by an itchy throat. As many others would, I had assumed that it was just 'one of those things' which one puts up with rather than bother one's doctor with such silly trivia.
>
> I followed the diet and bought some garlic pills. Its effects had immediate results. I could eat without fearing some after effects, I didn't itch as much and what is more my elbows had almost recovered their normal appearance. In fact my elbows became a useful yardstick against which

to assess how offensive the yeast was; I could almost 'clean them up' like a board and judge the damage within an hour of eating. Hard blotchy bits of skin would form, followed by itching, which would subside once more when I took some garlic pills.

I went back to my nutritionist, piecing together the relevant details, finding new ones even, such as my premature birth and being fed sugared water. I also remembered the numerous stomach upsets of my childhood and the nickname 'Chink' because of my jaundiced complexion.

I next interviewed Gwen in 1989. Eighteen months previously she had decided that she needed a career change, and had systematically looked for a therapy which she could train in that combined emotional release with physical awareness. Although her logical need was to find another career, she recognises that intuitively she was also looking for something to help her resolve her physical problems and their underlying emotional triggers.

In the Gerda Boyesen method it's up to the client – if you can't express yourself verbally then they can work on the body, using massage. It's the constant shift from one to the other which makes you progress. Plus the space and time they give you that is important. You actually feel that you can lean on someone, and allow yourself to feel and accept the weaknesses that you have. Normally you don't allow yourself to feel the things that hurt you because you don't have the resources to do it unsupported. The theory is that all psychological problems get lodged somewhere in the body through a build-up of hormonal byproducts. You begin to understand more and more as memories come into your mind. But you're the one in charge doing the work.

I used to live in my head. Now I live in the rest of my body as well. The therapist constantly asks me what is happening in my body. I resisted finding out at first. But you begin to feel the connection between the gut and emotion. When you come to feel your body as self-regulating, you begin to get a response to your biochemical problems as well. This came about through actually listening to my body and its needs, which is what I'd never done. I used to stuff myself with anything, and my gut gave up. Looking at the X-rays, done when I was in my teens, my gut was like a potato sack.

I was an unwanted baby, born when my mother was 42. As a child I didn't eat, then one bright day we went on holiday and my father held my hand. From that day onwards I started eating. My childhood was such a horrendous story of having to avoid being beaten or told off. I was never allowed to make any choices. My life wasn't my own to decide. It was the same with my gut. I hadn't learnt to discriminate between what I put into it, because I didn't value myself. No one did. I just functioned like a robot.

For me the big breakthrough was discovering that I have a choice as an adult. As a child the alternatives were far too threatening, life threatening, had I chosen not to obey. Anger is still a problem for me. I wasn't allowed to have tantrums. I'm having them now in therapy.

The other helpful thing that I did was a short self-assertiveness course. There was one sentence that made a deep impression on me. We were told that guilt doesn't belong to you. It is passed on to you, and you can choose to take it on board or throw it off.

Discovering the diagnosis of candida was important because I found the physical root. I got to the psychological problems later because it's too hard when you feel yourself the victim to be told on top of that 'Well, my dear, you've got psychological problems.' So you can use the physiological problems as a lever to try and sort yourself out. I was told it was all in my mind, but it was said in such a dismissive way. Added on the end should have been 'That's great, because change is possible. Yes, you do have a choice.' You can re-programme your mind, gain some self-esteem. Only you can decide to change your patterns. You don't need a doctor for that.

After the breakdown of my marriage I was at a point where I could not let go of anything. I had to be ill because I had to force myself to ask for outside help. I was so alone and somehow it was easier to be ill than to go mad with hurt.

Gwen's symptoms have all gone, except for small patches of psoriasis, and a continuing difficulty with alcohol, which she feels is no bad thing. She follows the Hay diet, whereby proteins and carbohydrates are not mixed, and eats well. Her life has a new purpose, because of the satisfaction she gains from treating clients through massage. She feels that her 12 years of studying linguistics is linked to the fact that her mother was unable to communicate verbally. Leaving that behind her has allowed her to move from the intellectual to the more intuitive, feeling and creative side of her personality.

17
CASE HISTORIES – MEN

Mike's and Steve's stories are presented here because of the persistent presence of candida from early on, and the failure on the part of doctors to provide appropriate treatment.

MIKE

Mike is 29, single and living on his own. His health problems started with allergic reactions in childhood and thrush in his adolescence. With hindsight he recognises that his mistreated candida was part of a general failing of his immunity, which has now left him with ME.

He worked as a mathematician and computer programmer, utilising computer graphics in pharmaceutical research. Before he was forced to give up work he was earning a good salary. He tried for a long time to carry on working, afraid of unemployment and feeling pressure from his family to carry on because they did not fully understand the extent of his symptoms. Both parents had experienced unemployment and were proud of their son's academic success. An unsympathetic GP refused to put ME on his sick certificate, preferring 'exhaustion' instead.

In his teens he had many bouts of thrush, including a rash on his genitals. He was always itching. He remembers that his diet as a child had not been good, and at university he lived on chocolate bars and junk food. Chocolate seemed to give him energy, but for the rest of the time he was often tired.

A year after leaving university he developed a rash all over his body, for which he was given a steroid cream. Eventually a specialist diagnosed a systemic yeast infection. He was prescribed the antifungal drug Nizoral for two months. The condition cleared but came back within six months.

In his mid-20s he caught what he describes as a viral

infection. Heavily involved in playing percussion in a band after work, he carried on, both at work and in the band. Left two weeks later with a sore throat, dizziness and problems of balance, his GP put him on three courses of antibiotics and some travel sickness pills. His symptoms worsened and increased to include blocked ears, aching glands and extreme fatigue.

Finally he was forced to give up what he loved most – he sold his drum kit to resist the temptation to play. Every time he played he needed time off work to recover. A new GP gave him monthly courses of antibiotics, and that year he went into hospital five times for urological operations. His thrush problems returned, and his tolerance for physical exercise plummeted.

Eventually he read about clinical ecology, and decided to consult a private doctor in nearby Manchester, who recognised allergies. He was tested for allergies, given nystatin and put on a yeast-free diet. Within a month he was significantly better, and after six he was almost back to normal. But it was to be a short respite, because soon after he caught chickenpox. He lost weight and was forced to seek help from friends.

> I felt extremely ill, was aching all over, couldn't think straight, had difficulty pronouncing words, and would often come out with undecipherable jibberish. I gave up living alone as I was too ill to look after myself, and I moved in for a few months with some good friends who lived nearby.

He realises that since taking nystatin he has had problems with his digestion.

> I have gastroenteritis all the time. I have to rest for half-an-hour after going to the loo. At one stage when I went to the loo I would itch for an hour afterwards. I'm worse on damp days, and living here it's always foggy and misty [Mike lives near Liverpool].

When he is out with friends he is tempted by sweet things, and takes more nystatin than usual as an antidote.

Mike found it difficult to penetrate the hurried consultations with his private doctor, and was unable to express his worries and fears for the future. Consulting a dermatologist on the National Health, he was told that he could not have a systemic yeast infection because he did not have other problems that accompany it, like skin rashes. Stool and blood tests confirmed the view that there was nothing wrong, and that he should come off the nystatin. But as soon as he came off nystatin his sore throat returned and his ears became blocked. Two weeks after leaving the hospital his rashes returned. His aching glands were dismissed because they did not appear swollen.

> She made me feel quite down. She made me think maybe I had been imagining it all this last year. Maybe nystatin was a placebo effect, so I stopped and went downhill and relapsed. Only this time I was worse. So I felt really bitter and angry about that woman. It's as though they won't take your word for it. I know nystatin was working, but I wanted to know why and I wanted to get to the root of the problem.
>
> I don't want my life to be taken over by my health. When you read about some people, their life is totally ruled by it. You can just become a hermit. It's antisocial to try and rotate diets. I try to live as normal a life as possible. I ought to get rid of my carpets because I'm allergic to house dust but I don't want to go to that extent. I want to feel normal, but I find it very difficult because I am forced to be aware of my symptoms.

Returning to his allergy doctor, Mike asked him how long it would be before he could play drums again. He said that Mike probably had ME, and that getting better was difficult because people with ME never regain their tolerance for exercise. This prognosis was devastating. He tried to find some satisfaction by forcing himself to achieve at work.

> But I pay for it afterwards. I feel quite happy when I'm productive. I'd really value my health if I had it back. I used to be a really high achiever, and now I'm scared of being put in a position where I can't compete with everyone else because of my illness.

Mike knows he has a problem about being assertive with doctors, and getting across the extent of his symptoms and his worries. He saw this lack of assertiveness at work also.

> It stems from my father, always knowing the right way to do things. He was forever stepping in. I laugh now. But I didn't when I was younger. You always feel one step down. I've never been able to talk to him. He felt a bit threatened by my education. He never said 'Well done.' He doesn't show

emotions. I didn't need to go into all this until I became ill and needed a solution. I feel all this might be relevant in some way.

I find it hard not being able to talk to my parents about my illness. It would be easier with cancer. You feel you would have something to show for packing up your job. My parents think I am perfectly normal. They think I'll snap out of it and get back to normal. They're embarrassed by illness.

Before giving up work Mike had gone to his GP, having written down his case history for her. He wanted her to write to his employers suggesting that he went part-time for six months.

As soon as I sat down I couldn't give her the case history. You don't have the nerve to say 'Look, I've been really ill with this. It's not just a sore throat.' You want to come right out with it, and you can't because there are ten people in the waiting room. I didn't give her the case history.

I feel quite inadequate. I wouldn't enter another relationship with anyone.

I wouldn't want to feel that I was the weaker one, like a nurse/patient relationship. I would rather stay on my own. At one point my doctor was saying that it was all stress. I just wouldn't wear that because at weekends I was noticeably worse because I used to go out and have a couple of drinks. I'm not a laid back person really. People say that I look it, but I'm not really. I worry about things. I used to feel an inner contentedness because of my abilities, but not any more.

After the interview, and after failing to keep up in a new job, Mike decided that he could no longer carry on working. He recognised that his difficulty in making himself rest was not helping him get better. Perhaps admitting he is ill enough not to work will allow him to meet his own needs, rather than try against all the odds to carry on pretending that his illness is less debilitating than it really is. The problem is that without work he is more cut-off and isolated.

STEVE

Steve, aged 50, lives with his wife and two children. Because of ME he has taken early retirement from his job as a teacher of social work in a college of further education.

Until he had ME in his late 40s he had never heard of candidiasis. At a conference on ME one of the speakers mentioned a symptom that he had had since he was 20 – an itchy bottom or anal thrush. From that point he connected other symptoms that he had, such as stomach bloating, a bad taste in his mouth, irritable bowel syndrome, migraines and sugar craving. Over the years attempts to present these symptoms to the GP had not led to any resolution, except the suggestion that he sort out his personal problems.

He describes himself as always a very anxious child, partly because he was born at the beginning of the war and was evacuated from London twice.

> I suppose I am rewriting my own history now because I used to see my earlier health problems as my mother encouraging illness, but thinking back I was actually ill. I had lots of sore throats. At nine or ten I saw a specialist for headaches, and I used to get one bout of viruses a year which would last a long time.

At 16 he developed a phobia about cancer, and eventually in his mid-20s he went into group therapy in an attempt to look at the underlying causes of his depression.

His diet when he was younger was mostly junk food, eaten very quickly with little ceremony. He always hated milk. He remembers being forced by his parents to drink Milk of Magnesia because of his stomach problems. Whenever he was ill he was given milky food.

After his marriage his digestive difficulties improved. But until he lost weight with ME, he was overweight. Although he always hated being fat he was never able to lose weight.

Before marriage at 28 he had had many different jobs, interspersed with periods of unemployment. He recognises now how his mood swings, and their seasonal connection, affected his work.

> All this I realise now was literally linked with mood. I would be doing very well in a job when in my 'manic' mood. Then I'd get the sack at the beginning of spring when I would get depressed and change and be very anti-authority. I was a chef, a milkman, a salesman, worked in various offices and at Fords.

His experience with therapy and psychiatrists motivated him to take up social work training, and by the 1970s he was manager of a social services team in inner London. Moving out of social work into training was an attempt to cut down the stress levels after a 'mini-breakdown'. Personal therapy helped, but he was still left with generalised anxieties which seemed to get worse.

Steve had many periods of taking antibiotics. When he was 25 he developed a sore throat which lasted three months, and was prescribed three courses of antibiotics. His anal thrush increased.

Steve developed ME at Christmas 1987, after a period of stress in the family because of three deaths, and after he caught flu. It also happened to be his 'manic' period, the time of the year when it was very difficult to relax because of seemingly boundless creative energy. He was prescribed antibiotics for flu, but six weeks later he was no nearer going back to work. He decided to consult a private doctor who was medical adviser to the ME Association.

> I had already read about ME in *Here's Health*, but he said the article was nonsense and to take no notice of it because it talked about candida, vitamins and amino acids. He said these people must have shares in the vitamin companies and were to be ignored. (By this point I was beginning to wonder whether GPs had shares in the manufacturers of antibiotics.) He gave me a muscle biopsy which was extremely painful, and I'm not sure that I ever found out what it revealed.

When Steve asked about his stomach problems he was told that it was the virus, but was confirmed in his suspicion that that could not be the total explanation because coming off certain foods helped enormously, suggesting that allergies were involved. Following the candida diet seemed to help.

Transferring to another doctor, he chose one who recognised candida as part of ME. He was put on nystatin, and took vitamins and minerals. After a few weeks he started to feel better, but a very bad relapse occurred when he was forced to walk to a concert in which his daughter was singing, when the coach dropped him a quarter of a mile away. He lost the use of his legs for two weeks.

After developing prostatism, he decided to have colonic

irrigation. Seven colonics cured his itchy bottom, and helped the prostate problem.

Steve was given enzyme potentiated desensitisation, and at the time of our interview had had 11 or 12 treatments. He found it difficult to come off nystatin, but managed later on to reduce the dose and try without it for one week at a time. This was his own initiative, rather than his doctor's.

> EPD has helped, though I've had some bad side effects. After the fifth one I was rolling around on the floor for a week, feeling suicidal. I feel the doctors who give EPD should be more open about the side effects.

Despite his reservations he stuck with it, and has started to feel more energy in the mornings as a result, he feels, of EPD. However, at one stage he became allergic to everything except lamb and tapioca.

Steve feels that he has had a positive view of the future since his bad experience with EPD, which he sees as a turning point. He is relieved to realise that his depressions have gone, along with the anxiety that came with them.

> Since I went on the diet and the anti-candida treatment, I haven't been depressed. So I've got a very strange relationship with ME, because I'd rather have ME than depression. All my memories of summer are of fighting depression. It has been suggested to me that my depression was possibly triggered by pollen in spring.

Although his mental symptoms have gone, he is still very limited in how far he can walk. When his legs stopped aching, he tried extending his walking by a few steps each day, but five days later his knees locked, and sleep was interrupted by aching and throbbing muscles. He still cannot drive.

He worries about the effect of his illness on his family, and the burden on his wife, who now works full-time as well as taking on most of the household chores. However his wife assures him that he is a 'different person' because his depressions have gone and he is more outgoing. Despite the limitations on Steve's life because of his restricted mobility, he is grateful for the chance to give up the pressures of full-time work and to get to know his children in a new way. His time is not wasted while at home because of his voluntary work as a 'listening ear' for other ME sufferers who need counselling, and his involvement in the 'politics' of ME.

The contrast with Mike's position is striking. By taking the courageous step of finally allowing himself to give up work, Mike committed himself to isolation at home. The lack of acceptance or understanding of his condition from his family, and the pessimism and limited concern of doctors, does not provide the support and encouragement that he needs.

18 DIAGNOSIS AND FINDING HELP

Labelling symptoms does not necessarily get to the bottom of the problem. For example, hypoglycaemia as a diagnosis does not answer the question why that particular person cannot handle sugar. However, most people are greatly relieved to have a name for their problem, especially with candidiasis, because of the difficulty within conventional medicine of getting recognition.

DIAGNOSIS AND HELP

If you think you have candidiasis, and if you are unable to get a sympathetic response from your GP, the simplest way to confirm your suspicions is to complete one of the candida questionnaires in this and many other books on candida (see pages 184–5). One of the objections to candida is that its symptoms are too numerous and too common, thus allowing anxious and neurotic individuals to jump on the bandwagon and demand attention for something that may have other causes. One way to overcome this danger is to ask your doctor to make some suggestions as to the cause of your symptoms, and then, if there is no satisfactory answer, or if all the tests come back negative when you know there is something wrong, it will do no harm to start by following an anti-candida diet.

Although many of the interviewees showed the value of taking control, no one managed to help themselves in total isolation. We all need outside support and encouragement, and many of the therapies available are positive aids at building immunity and fostering change.

But finding an alternative practitioner or doctor with experience of candidiasis usually means having the resources to pay, unless you have the patience to wait to see one of the few NHS doctors who specialise in allergies and food intolerance. Even then the treatment offered may be no more than diet, nystatin and EPD.

If you feel you have no choice but to pay for your treatment, you should be aware that many private practitioners and doctors sell what they prescribe, and consequently gain 25 per cent commission from the suppliers and manufacturers. Even if you buy straight from the manufacturer, using a 'prescription' from your practitioner, some companies still pay 25 per cent of total sales to the prescriber each month. This practice may be acceptable if the fees you are paying are correspondingly low. But linking prescribing habits with financial gain is not in the interests of the consumer. However, I know of one private clinical ecologist, and there may be others, who set aside time to write in detail to his patients' NHS doctors, explaining the symptoms and asking them to prescribe what is needed, so that patients do not have to pay more than his fees. He does not carry any stock himself, but has made arrangements with a local chemist to ensure that he stocks what his patients may be forced to buy if their NHS doctor refuses to prescribe.

One way to find a practitioner who recognises candidiasis is to join a self-help group and talk to others who have benefited from a consultation. This is easier for those with ME because the ME Association and the ME Action Campaign have local groups where contact is possible. Whether private or state funded, finding a practitioner who is prepared to listen fully is very important.

You may find that you get just as much support and help from practitioners who are not medically qualified but are trained in other areas such as nutrition, acupuncture, kinesiology, etc. In a situation where demand for help is not being met, new services are constantly being offered to meet the need. Erica, one of the interviewees, found that more and more people were ringing and asking her for advice, and eventually she was able to supply them with vitamins and minerals and antifungal treatments like Capricin and Allicin Complex. Her ongoing training as a nutritional counsellor was useful, but almost as important was her ability to offer clients telephone contact for the time when they most needed support.

This is a necessary service. In contrast, one doctor who specialises in ME ensures that patients only telephone when they are desperate by charging them £25 for fifteen minutes.

This may be an effective way of organising time, but certainly inhibits patients when they need help because of the distressing effects of 'die-off' or of treatments such as enzyme potentiated desensitisation.

Some practitioners may combine skills. For example, finding a psychotherapist who is also aware of the importance of nutrition is an effective way of getting a broader perspective.

TESTS FOR CANDIDIASIS

None of the interviewees in the book had a test at the outset to confirm the fact that they had candidiasis. But tests do exist and are being developed. Thus Carol was given the dark-field test by Dr Erdmann, which claims to show candida byproducts, if present systemically, in a live blood sample. Dr Erdmann also has a urine test to identify the presence of yeast and missing digestive enzymes. Samples can be sent to Bioscreen for analysis. In America Dr Elias Ilyia, co-developer of the Jarvik artificial heart, has developed the Candascan test based on a stool culture. The test evaluates what are normal and abnormal levels of candida, and whether the mycelial form is present. This test is not available in the UK, but one company is considering plans to import it.

The Legarde test is a diagnostic test for cancer. Using whole blood looked at through a microscope, it also shows the invasion of toxic products from systemic candida, and viral activity. It has been used extensively by immunologists Dr Gerlac and Dr Issels in West Germany and is now available in this country. But the symptom checklist, and diagnosis on the basis of improvement after treatment, is for the moment the most accessible way to find out if you have candida.

ME sufferers also rely on a careful history, and the exclusion of other conditions. An enterovirus test is available at St Mary's Hospital, London, but although a positive test indicates the presence of enterovirus in the blood, it is not a reliable test for ME because a negative result does not exclude the diagnosis of ME.

The danger of relying on a test for antiviral activity as an indicator of ME is that such tests may come to assume more importance than an assessment of all the cofactors that cause the illness.

MISTAKEN DIAGNOSES

Even if your symptoms lead you to believe that you have candida or ME, there are certain conditions that could mislead you into a wrong diagnosis or which might be present as well.

Dr Leo Galland suggests that intestinal parasites are a common cause of problems such as diarrhoea, colitis and dysentery, extra-intestinal tissue invasion, irritable bowel syndrome, bloating and malabsorption. Other frequent symptoms are food intolerance and food allergy, and rheumatic symptoms, together with chronic fatigue and night sweats.

The commonest parasites found in the United States, the United Kingdom and Australia are protozoa (one-celled animals), particularly *Giardia lamblia* (an intestinal parasite) and *Entamoeba histolytica* (typically associated with amoebic dysentery). The development of AIDS was preceded in the gay community by an epidemic of intestinal parasites, further reducing immune function because of the large amounts of drugs taken to treat them. Dr Galland found an unacceptably high level of false negatives from routine and purged stool examination, and has developed instead a test using rectal mucus. Dr Galland claims successful treatment with a herb called *Artemisia annua*. Black walnut tea is also effective. Herbs used in conjunction with colonic irrigation have been particularly successful as a way of treating parasites.

19
ROOTING IT OUT

When discussing treatment for candidiasis it is important to emphasise that there is no one way that is applicable to everyone; the case studies are clear evidence of that. We all have different biochemical needs and different constellations and chronicity of symptoms. To see disease as a function of the cause misses the more accurate view that its manifestation depends on the host response, which is always different.

Having made the point that we are all different, it is also necessary to emphasise our shared ability to activate the body's own healing potential. Finding the right way for your needs is sometimes a process of trial and error. Having the determination and persistence, despite ill health, depends on a fundamental optimism that balance is possible. Underneath it all, then, is the recognition of our own value and right to exist. The following sections provide information and advice on diet, antifungal supplements and nutrition. A bibliography at the end of the book (pages 184–5) is given for those who wish to go into greater detail.

Nystatin is the treatment of choice for many doctors who treat candidiasis. In an article sponsored by Lambert's, makers of nutritional supplements, Dr Belinda Dawes, when discussing candida, takes the view that 'six weeks on a low carbohydrate diet is usually enough to starve the yeast out of the system'. But this view is optimistic and fails to take account of underlying imbalances and problems. Her book, with Dr Damien Downing, also recommends nystatin and Mycocidin, together with nutritional supplements. Dr Brostoff recommends a course of nystatin for at least two months. Yet some of the case studies in this book were on nystatin for at least two years because they found that discontinuing nystatin only brought their symptoms back with increased severity. This chapter will argue that the effect of nystatin on candida can be likened to a lawnmower, slicing off the top, but leaving the fungal roots unaffected and in a better position to proliferate.

Moreover, the standard use of nutritional supplements to accompany an antifungal drug like nystatin does not guarantee that what is taken in will not be excreted out. Most people who have problems with candidiasis are malabsorbers. By avoiding food and chemical allergies at the start of anti-candida treatment, and thereby taking the load off the immune system, and by replacing missing digestive enzymes, the body is better able to digest and absorb.

Diet is important, but many sufferers find that it is not usually possible to control candida by diet alone. Thus, if the candida is outside the gastrointestinal tract, a low sugar diet will not be effective on its own because candida can extract sugar from blood circulating in the bloodstream. Mycopryl, garlic, digestive enzymes, allergy avoidance, nutritional supplementation and repopulation of the gut with beneficial bacteria are also essential partners in any such treatment regime.

One of the difficulties with following restrictive diets is that the motivation to stick to them is in direct relationship to the severity of your symptoms and your need to overcome them. If your candidiasis is long-standing and chronic, finding the motivation to follow the diet will not be too difficult at first, although finding the staying power to make fundamental change is never easy.

However, diet alone is not recommended. Many candida sufferers need to address long-standing problems of malabsorption; sticking rigidly to a diet will not necessarily bring long-term relief, and may lead to disillusion and failure.

FOODS TO AVOID

Sugar

All carbohydrates we eat eventually end up as glucose and other simple sugars circulating in the bloodstream, these being the basic building blocks of carbohydrate metabolism. However, complex carbohydrates take some time, and a number of chains of enzymatic reactions, before they become degraded to glucose. In contrast, sugar and other simple carbohydrates are broken down very quickly in the gut. The glucose is then absorbed and floods into the bloodstream, where it is circulated to the rest of the body and absorbed by the cells, to be used as a fuel or stored.

The level of circulating glucose in the bloodstream is controlled by a hormone called insulin, produced in the pancreas; it is insulin that allows and regulates the passage of glucose out of the bloodstream and into the cells. Insulin is produced in response to the presence of glucose in the blood. Stimulant drinks containing caffeine (tea, coffee, cola drinks) can also induce the same response; they produce a flood of glucose from the liver (a storage organ, among other things), resulting in a concomitant surge of insulin.

So a typical sugar-rich western diet, apart from directly encouraging yeast overgrowth, gives us large peaks and troughs in the levels of blood sugar, as glucose floods into the bloodstream after a meal or snack and is then removed under the influence of a corresponding peak of insulin. As a corollary, a diet rich in sugar is likely to be low in important nutrients, minerals and vitamins. The result of these wild fluctuations in blood sugar levels coupled with a poor overall diet is that, over time, the health and even the character of the individual can be affected. The endocrine glands may operate less efficiently, causing hormone imbalances and altered body chemistry. The immune system can be compromised, giving less efficient clearance of infections and other complications. And the erratic overloading of the insulin-producing cells in the pancreas can cause them to function less efficiently, resulting in a vicious spiral of cause and effect. It is surely no coincidence that pancreatic deficiency is often found in candidiasis sufferers.

All forms of sugar should therefore be excluded from the diet, including honey, molasses, maple syrup, sugar substitutes, quick acting carbohydrates and all alcoholic drinks. Milk sugar (lactose) from milk products should also be cut out. In the beginning it may be wise to cut out fruit sugar – pineapple, grapefruit, lemon and avocado are among the few permissible fruits. Later on more fruits can be gradually reintroduced. And remember that many foods have 'hidden sugar'; frozen peas, most canned foods and many packaged foods have sugar added to them as part of their processing, and should be avoided.

Gluten

Dr Nadya Coates, director of the Springhill Cancer Centre, overcame and controlled leukaemia and liver cancer by following, as one of her treatment protocols, an anti-candida diet. Her view is that cancer will not appear unless candida infection is extensive in the small intestine.

One of the food constituents that she recommends candida sufferers to avoid is gluten, found in wheat and, to a lesser extent, rye, oats and barley. Oatbran and oatgerm are free of gluten as the gluten occurs in the centre of the oat. Millet, rice and corn are completely gluten free.

Gluten is a sticky viscous protein which can be recognised as an allergen by the body, particularly if there are deficiencies of certain antibodies in the gut in the first year of life (as a result, it would appear, of not being breastfed). Furthermore, the gluten-containing food particles can become coated with fungal organisms if candida is present, preventing the particles from being digested and allowing them to build up as deposits of hardened sticky food, mucus and fungi on the gut wall, affecting absorption of other nutrients. These deposits can then act as foci for other microorganisms, leading to putrefaction and the subsequent production of harmful waste and byproducts. And of course this ignores the fact that the gluten-containing food particles will be lost as a source of nutrients.

As a side issue, genetic engineering of grains has increased their gluten content and made them more permeable to fungal and environmental toxins. In this respect, wheat, barley and rye have the weakest protective husks, whereas oats are the least permeable.

Most anti-candida diets cut out bread because of the sugar used to activate the yeast in the baking of bread, and the yeast itself. The need for further restrictions of all gluten-containing grains may seem difficult, but the pay-off in terms of greater energy and well being make such deprivations easier to tolerate. However, it should be borne in mind that strict adherence to a gluten-free diet, whilst necessary for those trying to overcome a terminal disease, may not seem so easy when you are already adjusting to the normal anti-candida diet and when your symptoms are not so severe.

As with any 'advice', it is important to arm yourself with knowledge and then work out what is possible for you, within your own aspirations and capabilities. One compromise could be to cut out wheat, barley and rye entirely, but to have oats. Oatbran fibre added to food is also a good way to increase the absorptive surface of faecal material, an important consideration when trying to rid the body of dead candida cells.

Yeast and mould-containing foods

Tolerance for yeast products and mould varies. It is wise to cut out bread, vinegar, mushrooms, cheeses, spices and condiments, alcohol, fruit and fruit juices, dried fruit, all malted products, all foods containing monosodium glutamate, peanuts and pistachios, all other nuts when they're not fresh, processed and cooked meats, left-over food, tea, coffee and herbal teas. However, one herbal tea that is recommended is Taheebo tea or Pau D'Arco tea, because of its antifungal properties.

Even if at a later stage you find that you can tolerate yeast, Dr Crook warns that alcoholic drinks contain large amounts of quick-acting carbohydrate which provide nourishment for candida.

Milk

Apart from the need to avoid milk sugar, pasteurised milk should not be consumed because it encourages candida overgrowth. However Dr Crook does not suggest cutting out butter.

Carbohydrates

Any carbohydrates which have been refined beyond the simple grinding stage are undesirable. In the early days it was thought that a low carbohydrate diet was necessary, and some practitioners still recommend a very low intake of carbohydrates if the rest of the diet is ineffective. However, taking digestive enzymes and using an effective antifungal agent like Capricin should obviate the need to cut out carbohydrates, which for some people leads to too much weight loss and unsatisfied hunger.

FOODS TO EAT

Foods that you can eat include fresh vegetables, small amounts of fruit gradually introduced after a few weeks, fresh nuts, seeds, beans, grains (millet, rice and corn are gluten-free), yogurt, eggs, fresh meats (except beef and pork) and all seafood. Two 'new' cereals, both from South America, are amaranth and quinoa; they are both low in gluten, and have a high protein content.

Many people worry about calcium deficiency upon giving up milk, but sesame seeds have twice as much calcium as milk, while pumpkin seeds contain up to 30 per cent protein and are a good source of zinc. Dry-roasted pumpkin seeds, together with sunflower seeds, make a good and nutritious snack.

The anti-candida diet recommends high protein levels. However, animal protein is difficult to digest, and, unless organic, is often laced with hormones and antibiotics (lamb, rabbit and wild game are less likely to be affected). Dr Coates recommends breaking down animal protein as much as possible by marinating meat in lemon juice, or cooking it with onions, garlic or yogurt. Supplementation with vegetable enzymes also helps. When buying chicken it is safer to choose those that are corn fed as they are least exposed to fungal contamination.

Essential fatty acids

Just as glucose is one of the basic building blocks of carbohydrate metabolism, fatty acids are the basic building blocks of fats and oils and are particularly important constituents of cell membranes. Three of these fatty acids – linoleic acid, linolenic acid and arachidonic acid – are essential for growth, although only linoleic acid is absolutely essential in the diet as the other two can be synthesised from it. However, to maintain good health it is important that we obtain adequate amounts of all three in our diet. These essential fatty acids (EFAs) regulate many body processes, and a diet rich in EFAs is likely to protect the body against invasion from bacteria and viruses, and control candida by ensuring healthy cell membranes.

Linseed oil is the best known source of linolenic acid; one to two tablespoons of cold-pressed fresh linseed oil daily is recommended for candida sufferers. It should be sold in an opaque bottle or can and, once purchased, it should be stored in a cool dark place and used within three weeks. It can be added to hot food, or used instead of olive oil for salads or mayonnaise, but it should not be used for cooking because heat destroys its nutritional value. It is also available, emulsified, in stabilised capsules. Whole linseeds can be used as an alternative, but you need four times as many seeds to oil. Whole seeds are best, so that they can be freshly ground in a food blender and then added to cereals and other food. Other sources are spinach, green beans, kale, lettuce, parsley, green peppers and bean sprouts. Fish oils, present in salmon, trout, sardines and mackerel are also important sources of EFAs.

Hydrogenation, a process used in the manufacture of margarines, damages these fatty acids. Dr Erdmann recommends Vitaquell as the only safe margarine to use; your local healthfood shop should stock it.

As already explained, linoleic acid is essential for life and necessary for the manufacture of other fatty acids. The main dietary source for those with candida is safflower oil, brown rice, sweetcorn, avocados, pumpkin seeds, sunflower seeds and sesame seeds and oil. Once linoleic acid has been absorbed into the body, the next stage in the metabolic pathway to other fatty acids is its conversion to gammalinoleic acid (GLA), a process for which you need zinc, magnesium, vitamin B6 and biotin. Unfortunately, candida sufferers are usually deficient in these nutrients, so it is useful to supplement the diet with GLA itself, as well as sources of linoleic acid.

GLA can be routinely added to the diet as a supplement by using evening primrose oil or blackcurrant seed oil. A new and more concentrated source is to be found in GLA Complex, distributed by BioCare; it is combined with organically produced linseed oil, nitrogen packed and emulsified. Questions have been raised about the advisability of combining GLA and fish oil; it is therefore a good precaution to take them separately at different times of the day.

OTHER DIETARY ADVICE

Digestive enzymes

From day one of the change of diet it is advisable to take a digestive enzyme supplement. Such supplements help our own digestive enzymes break down food into usable nutrients, such as amino acids, and are thus of great value to candida sufferers. They may also prevent further allergic food reactions, and ensure that the diet is not too restrictive. Enzymes from a vegetable origin have a higher biological activity rate than animal enzymes because they operate over a wider range of pH, and do not oxidise as quickly.

It used to be thought that stomach acid degraded such ingested enzymes and made them ineffective, but Dr Erdmann states that modern measurement techniques show that this is not the case. More elaborate studies have been carried out by medical biologist, Dr Peter Rothschild.

Food quality

Vegetables should be fresh and, if possible, organically grown. Many supermarkets now sell organic vegetables. If you cannot afford to buy all your vegetables organically produced, you can compromise; for example, organic carrots and potatoes are usually not as expensive as some other organic vegetables. Resist the temptation to buy perfect looking non-organic vegetables in supermarkets – high standards and customer preference for 'eye-appeal' may mean that above average amounts of chemicals are used to produce such specimens. Vegetables produced for smaller outlets may be a safer bet.

Adding powdered vitamin C to the water when washing vegetables kills any mould that may be growing on them. And scrub the vegetables with a stiff brush rather than peeling them (if organic), assuming the peel is edible; important nutrients are often concentrated in the skin or peel. Nutrient loss can be further minimised if you grate, mash or purée the vegetables just before use. Steaming vegetables in small amounts of water is better than boiling, and don't forget that you can use vegetable water in soup stocks for maximum nutrition.

Of all the non-organic meats, lamb and wild game are the most likely to be free of chemicals. If you eat liver and kidney, it is preferable to pay more and buy them from organic sources as these organs act as filters and stores, and can contain higher concentrations of chemicals than other parts of the animal carcase. Experimenting with pulses as a way of varying your sources of protein is a good idea.

Rotate

There is basic agreement among practitioners for the need to rotate food in order to avoid acquiring new allergies. The same food should only be eaten four days apart, although you may find it possible to eat rice more frequently. In this way, too, you can detect which food is affecting you badly. New work on the efficacy of digestive enzymes is demonstrating that many of the problems with shifting allergies could be avoided by taking digestive enzyme supplements.

Better habits

Starting the day with a glass of tepid water with a squeeze of fresh lemon juice or dilute apple vinegar is an effective way to reduce any candida activity in the throat that has built up overnight.

Because many candida problems stem from deficiencies in the digestive process, it is worth taking steps to ensure that the way you eat maximises good digestion. Thus, chewing food thoroughly, at least 20 times, is important; enzymes present in the saliva are essential to the digestion of carbohydrates. Drinking with meals is not recommended. Small portions of food eaten frequently are better than large amounts, and keeping protein separate from starches and fruits is also a good idea.

And it goes without saying that birth control pills, antibiotics, steroids, hormones and immunosuppressant drugs should not be taken whilst on the anti-candida treatment programme. However, stopping some of these drugs suddenly, particularly steroids, is not a good idea; you may need advice on how to come off them gradually.

What to expect

One way to get over the psychological difficulty of following a restrictive diet is to stick to it strictly for the first week. Then, if you feel a major improvement in your symptoms, it will not be too difficult to carry on. Gradually, over time, other foods can be reintroduced. (Sugar, though, is not a necessary part of the diet and should be avoided indefinitely.)

However, many of the case studies confirmed the generally accepted view that changing the diet does not start an uninterrupted change for the better. Be warned that some symptoms will recur, and new ones will arise as toxic waste is eliminated from the body. This is where it is important to have the support of an understanding practitioner, who can assess which symptoms are part of the 'healing crisis' and which could be alleviated by further changes in diet or other therapeutic inputs.

A useful book on candida, which provides more detailed advice on diet and specific recommendations for those who are allergic to twentieth-century life, is *Candida* by Dr Luc de Schepper. Unlike other candida specialists, he advises that sufferers avoid cold and raw foods, because of their effect on the spleen (this view is derived from Chinese medicine). Generally, though, raw food is seen as beneficial because heating has not destroyed naturally occurring enzymes which can assist digestion. As with all recommendations, it is up to you to work out in practice what suits your condition best; just because some advice is conflicting does not mean that you should give up in despair.

MOULD

It is important to check where you live for mould, often found in bathrooms, kitchens and clothes cupboards; houseplants are another source of mould spores. If you notice that your symptoms are worse in autumn this may be because of the mould spores released from rotting leaves.

KILLING OFF AND BUILDING UP

Mycopryl

Caprylic acid is a short-chain saturated fatty acid, derived from coconut oil, with antifungal properties. It appears to act in the same way as the fatty acids produced by our normal bowel flora, which ordinarily control the growth of candida.

Caprylic acid is available in different formulations and under different brand names, but from practitioners' experiences the most effective is Mycopryl (formerly Capricin), a compound devised by Dr Torbin Neesby, a pharmaceutical biochemist specialising in the nutritional and medical use of short-chain fatty acids. Being a natural product, Mycopryl does not require a prescription.

Mycopryl is a high-potency compound bound with insoluble calcium to allow for timed release of the caprylic acid, making it effective against candida infestation in the colon (large intestine). Some other formulations of caprylic acid are bound with sodium; they are thus water soluble and are absorbed too quickly in the upper reaches of the small intestine before they can act against candida further down the digestive tract. Mycopryl is also lipid (fat) soluble,so that it is able to penetrate the lipoprotein cell membrane, facilitating its ability to eliminate both surface and intercellular candida. Recent research has demonstrated that Mycopryl does not compete with beneficial microorganisms.

Mycopryl should be taken before food. If the die-off is strong lower the dose or avoid Mycopryl altogether for 24 hours. Drink plenty of water to flush the system out during this early stage. ME sufferers may find its mode of action too strong, and should always start on a low doseage.

A new product has been developed, combining garlic, caprylic acid, butyric acid, and aloe vera. This has been devised specifically to avoid relapse after treatment with Mycopryl, and should be taken once a day for two to three months. Its action gives the immune system more time to recover, and greater healing of the intestinal wall. Colon Guard, or CG233, is available from the manufacturers of Mycopryl.

DIE-OFF AND THE ILEOCAECAL VALUE

Sometimes the body's ability to eliminate a large amount of dead candida cells and their toxins is weak. 'Die-off' is the term used to describe these problems; it refers to the common tendency for symptoms to worsen after successful anti-fungal treatment. Dr George T. Lewith in *Candida and Thrush* recommends temporarily lowering the dose of Mycopryl, or cutting it out altogether for 48 hours until the reaction has settled. He also suggests drinking plenty of water in order to help elimination.

Initially, some practitioners were using Mycopryl at too high a dosage, and as a result stopped using it because of unpleasant reactions. It is advisable not to start Mycopryl until a week or so after starting an anti-candida diet.

Doctors who use enzyme potentiated desensitisation (see page 165) are of the opinion that Capricin did not combine well with this treatment, and use nystatin instead. It is possible that using Mycopryl from the start of anti-candida treatment obviates the need for EPD later on. In any event, both nystatin and EPD are expensive alternatives, and the harmful effects of nystatin are only just coming to be recognised.

Luc de Schepper has found that almost all candida patients have an open ileocaecal valve, the valve which normally prevents faeces from backing up from the large intestine into the small intestine, where waste products could be absorbed into the bloodstream. Killing off the candida cells in the large intestine allows the dead yeast cells and toxins released from the disrupted cells to escape back into the small intestine through this open valve; they are then absorbed by the bloodstream and their action on the rest of the body causes the symptoms of die-off and brain fogginess.

Acupressure is a very effective means of closing the ileocaecal valve. You can test for a weak valve by using Applied Kinesiology – a series of specific muscle tests are related to a meridian (energy pathway) and its associated organ, gland or system. Massage and light touch on body reflex points and acupuncture points help to retrain the valve to function normally.

Garlic

Garlic has been shown to be an effective inhibitor of fungal growth, and should be a major part of any treatment against candida. However most garlic supplements have been found to be of minimal medicinal effect because allicin, the main anti-infective component of garlic, is easily denatured. Fresh garlic is always preferable. However freeze dried garlic has been found to be effective, particularly Blackmore's Garlix.

Oxy-Pro

Oxy-Pro utilises the fact that yeasts do not thrive in well-oxygenated cells. It is a potassium/sodium compound that releases oxygen at the site of application, thus having a direct effect on any microorganisms that might have colonised the area. (It is not to be confused with hydrogen peroxide.)

Oxy-Pro is good for the lymphatics, head, neck and chest regions, but not for the colon. If you have problems with your sinuses or ears this may help, as long as it is used in conjunction with the other treatments, thus ensuring that eradication is long-term. It can also be used as a mouthwash for oral thrush, applied topically to finger and toenails, used as a nasal douche and applied to the ear.

Aloe vera juice

Aloe vera juice is recommended by Leon Chaitow for its antifungal action, together with its beneficial effects on bowel flora. *Aloe vera* is a desert plant. It is claimed to be detoxifying, immune boosting, a useful healing aid and a good source of

EFAs. Apart from taking it internally, in juice form, it can be applied topically to fungal skin infections.

Biotin and oleic acid

The B vitamin biotin helps limit yeast's tendency to transform to the fungal form and, used together with *Lactobacillus acidophilus*, between meals, is an essential agent of control. Leon Chaitow warns that raw egg white should not be included in the anti-candida diet because it neutralises biotin's beneficial effect on the body.

Cold-pressed virgin olive oil contains a substance called oleic acid which has a similar effect on the yeast as biotin; six teaspoons a day, divided into three doses, with or without food, is recommended.

Colonics and enemas

Having starved and killed the yeast, the next task is to get rid of it. The build up of sticky mucus along the lining of the colon makes evacuation of dead yeast cells in the faeces less likely. Colonics and enemas are an effective way of dislodging such impacted material.

Enemas can be self administered, but are less effective than colonics because they cannot pass water up the whole length of the large intestine. Apart from water, it is possible to add to an enema ingredients such as acidophilus or Pau D'Arco tea; coffee enemas detoxify the liver, and BioCare have developed rectal implants of enzymes which help to dislodge entrenched mucus.

Colonics depend on the expertise of the colonic therapist. It is important that pre-sterilised disposable hoses and speculums are used, to avoid the danger of contamination. The colon is exercised by the water pressure, which stimulates the expansion and contraction of the muscular walls. Herbal implants can be used, as well as acidophilus products to introduce beneficial flora. Green Farm produce colon supplements which include bulking agents and herbal combinations. Colon Care from BioCare combines enzyme activators and psyllium for improved nutrient absorption and mucus removal.

Some people have short-term symptoms of nausea and diarrhoea after a colonic, so it is important to rest afterwards. Extreme cases of ME may be advised to wait before taking such an invasive treatment.

Probiotic supplementation

Replacing the indigenous flora in the gut is one way to boost your body's natural ability to keep unwanted microorganisms under control. *Lactobacillus acidophilus*, bifidobacteria and *Lactobacillus bulgaricus* are usually cultured from a milk base; until recently, other such products not cultured from a milk base were not as effective.

According to independent research scientists Drs Nigel Plummer and Sue Pinney, the best biologically active form of probiotic on the market is Bio-Acidophilus. Lamberts also market it under the name Super Acidophilus Plus. In this product enzyme-activated acid-stable bifidobacteria and acidophilus are combined. Although it is cultured from a milk-free base, it has the advantages of a milk-based culture because it is grown on enzyme-activated lactose (milk sugar). This enables those with lactose and milk intolerance to benefit from it, the enzymes substituting for the missing digestive enzymes in the gut. The fact that it's acid stable means that it's not degraded in the acid environment of the stomach and can be taken with food.

Some probiotics contain *Streptococcus faecium* and *Streptococcus faecalis*, found in the faeces of humans and animals and in insects and plants. However, until there is stronger evidence about the possible beneficial effects of these bacteria for humans it is wise to avoid using them. Studies are difficult because of the marked difference in response from individual to individual.

One week after starting Mycopryl it is advisable to start repopulating the gut. Taking a probiotic straight away would not be sensible because the toxins from die off in the first week would overwhelm the beneficial bacteria. And avoid products which are tableted; some of the bacteria are destroyed by the heat generated during the tableting process.

Butyric acid and Enteroplex

Butyric acid is recommended in order to heal the gut wall. It is a short chain fatty acid found in butter and olive oil, and is produced in a healthy gut by the fermentation of undigested carbohydrates and fibres by friendly anaerobic bacteria (bacteria that function in the absence of oxygen). Apart from its effectiveness at healing damaged mucosa, it is also a beneficial anti-cancer food because it helps produce interferon.

Enteroplex is a vitamin U extract derived from cabbage juice. It is mildly anti-fungal, and research shows that it increases the amount of friendly bacteria by 10–12 per cent.

Vitamins and minerals

Individual needs for vitamins and minerals vary enormously, and testing by hair, sweat and serum analysis is important. Because treating the candida problem may resolve some of the vitamin and mineral deficiencies that accompany candida, it may be sensible to wait to be tested until after a few weeks of the candida treatment. And always remember that any supplements you take should be yeast free.

Magnesium, working with calcium, is important for muscle function, regular heart rhythm, and mood. Magnesium is also involved in many enzyme systems and chemical reactions. The richest dietary sources of magnesium are also the richest dietary sources of essential fatty acids, such as seedfoods and fish. Dolomite tablets combine magnesium and calcium, but they are relatively unabsorbable and may be contaminated with toxic metals, so that most good nutritionists do not recommend them. Synthetic magnesium, in the form of magnesium acetate, has been used by some nutritionists, but reports of effects on the liver and blood are not encouraging; it may be wise to avoid this product until further studies confirm or deny its beneficial effects. Magnesium aspartate and magnesium citrate are good sources.

However Dr Galland, in an interview with Dr Crook, states that yeast infections play havoc with the way magnesium is absorbed in the gut, largely because such an infection creates a deficiency of vitamin B6, upon which the absorption of magnesium is dependent. Thus supplementation alone may not cure the problem; getting to grips with candida could be more helpful.

Candida sufferers are usually also short of zinc, vitamin A and vitamin B3. The late Dr Carl Pfeiffer, who ran the Brain Bio Center in Princeton, New Jersey, has written extensively about 'pyroluria', whereby zinc and vitamin B6 are excreted in the urine. This can result in physical and psychological problems, and is stabilised by adequate supplementation. Supplementation of individual B vitamins, without a B complex, is not recommended because they all work synergistically.

Zinc is essential for the healthy production of T cells in the thymus. Supplementation away from food, because it is better absorbed, is usually recommended. Zinc citrate is more expensive but used more efficiently by the body; it is the form found in breast milk. Unfortunately some multivitamin and mineral tablets contain the cheaper and inferior zinc gluconate and zinc orotate. Natural sources of zinc are steak, lamb, pork, pumpkin seeds, eggs, mustard, soyabeans, turkey, most nuts, peas and berries.

Other vitamins that you may almost certainly benefit from are vitamin C, a powerful immune booster, and vitamin E, a strong antioxidant (defender of the cell membrane). Vitamin E works best when taken together with selenium.

Other supplements – beware

As awareness of candidiasis slowly increases, more supplements are appearing on the market. However, not all are as beneficial as they might seem to be.

Mycocidin is ranked with Capricin (now Mycopryl) as a 'natural retarder' by Drs Belinda Dawes and Damien Downing, and the manufacturers recommend nine to twelve tablets to be taken each day. A company owned by Dr Downing distributes Mycocidin in Britain. The label claims that this product is castor bean oil concentrate, but independent analysis on unmarked samples revealed that 11·6 per cent of each capsule was undecylenic acid, a synthetic substance produced by mixing and heating a catalyst with castor bean oil, and the remainder was olive oil. Undecylenic acid is not approved by the FDA in America for oral use, but is allowed to be used externally as a foot powder. It is toxic internally, and corrosive to the gastrointestinal mucosa.

Some manufacturers are seizing the initiative and marketing candida packs of tablets and capsules, combining different antifungal ingredients which are recommended to be taken at the same time. However, such combinations may not provide the correct potency for each substance, allowing candida the chance to continue to grow. Moreover, attempts to combine garlic with probiotics are of little proven value. Any combination formula containing caprylic acid should make sure that the caprylic acid is time-released. Binding the caprylic acid with sodium does not ensure that candida in the gut is reached, because it is absorbed too quickly in the stomach.

Vaginal thrush

Some women, despite following the candida programme, fail to totally free themselves of vaginal thrush. Two products are worth trying. Cervagyn cream can provide relief of minor vaginal irritations. It contains 3% potassium sorbate, combined with olive oil and camomile. In women with yeast infections only, continued application of this cream for 7–14 days removes the symptoms of swelling, itching and discharge. The pessary Cervagyn Plus, which combines Caprylic acid and lactobacillus, is another option for treating deeply embedded candida.

OTHER TREATMENTS

Nystatin

If you consult a doctor who recognises candidiasis, it may be suggested, if diet does not work on its own, that you take an antifungal drug. The number one choice is usually nystatin.

Nystatin is an antifungal antibiotic which is believed to kill or stop the growth of a limited number of strains of yeasts and yeast-like fungi. It is not thought to affect bacteria. It is described as unusually safe by Dr Crook because it is believed to be non-toxic and non-sensitising, even on prolonged administration. This is because, he argues, very little is absorbed from the intestinal tract. Although the initial reactions are often severe, this is not necessarily a reaction to the drug but the die-off or Herxheimer effect of dead yeast cells and their toxins. But, if we accept the view that those with candidiasis have a 'leaky gut' we should also be cautious about claims for the safety of nystatin because of its non-permeability.

Moreover some yeasts are embedded too deep in the wall of the mucous membrane of the gut wall to be reached by nystatin. It is unfortunate that many candida sufferers are advised to continue nystatin for some time to ensure that all the candida is destroyed when this is patently not possible if the candida is not one of the specific strains killed by nystatin, or if it is systemic. Dr Truss suggests that if exposure of the white blood cells to yeast products is reduced, they can begin to recover their ability to defend against fungal invasion on their own. But recovery by this route can take a long time, ignores the possible dangers of nystatin, and risks the sufferer giving up the diet in despair because of the length of time it takes to get results.

This split, between the belief in nystatin's safety and effectiveness and clear evidence in practice that long-term relief is not always found, is illustrated in an otherwise useful and informed book. Trowbridge and Walker in the *The Yeast Syndrome* describe nystatin favourably in the section devoted to it, with the proviso that it needs to be combined with other holistic methods. Yet, tucked away in another section on polyene antibiotics (one of which is nystatin), they refer to one study which suggests that nystatin may induce an increase in the number of colony-forming units of yeast cells.

> Researchers reported that the normally yeast-killing polyene antibiotics were bound to the fatty acids in the cell wall of the fungi, but they produced no toxic effect and actually stimulated the yeasts to increase the number of their colonies. No matter what the intended effect of antibiotics, they all hold the prospect of making our lives more difficult – even the ones we often rely on to help eradicate the yeast syndrome.

Clearly more research is needed. Some practitioners specialising in candidiasis are of the opinion that nystatin damages the sodium pump inside cells, pushing potassium out of the body. Whatever the basis of this view, it is surely worth detailed investigation, but whether we can expect the drug companies to initiate research is another matter. For the moment, too many prescriptions are being written to suggest the need for re-evaluation. If you find that coming off nystatin brings back your symptoms, it is advisable to combine nystatin with Mycopryl first, and gradually reduce your dose over time.

Amphotericin B

This drug is related to nystatin, and some doctors argue that it is more effective and better tolerated than nystatin. It is about one-third of the cost of nystatin. The French form of fungizone is thought to be preferable to the fungilin tablets and lozenges available in this country, because it provides a stronger, more effective dose and is in capsule form.

Although it can be bought over the counter in France, concern about potential side effects of fungizone has resulted in a ban on its use in the United States, although the more toxic form of intravenous amphotericin B is permissible if administered in a hospital. Dr Luc de Schepper has used fungizone when working in Europe, without noticing any side effects, and describes it as superior to nystatin. This is because amphotericin B is thought to be more effective at destroying candida cells which are buried deeper in the gut wall. Like nystatin, however, it is not effective systemically.

As already stated, given intravenously it is very toxic, but in oral use studies have concluded that it is safe. As with nystatin, views about its safety should be looked at cautiously, because of the possibility of absorption through the gut wall. *Meeting Place*, the periodical of The Australian and New Zealand Myalgic Encephalomyelitis Society (ANZYMES) in its Summer/Winter 1987–88 edition, reports one doctor's varied experience in using amphotericin B with his patients. Some people do very well with the drug, and it enables others to reduce their dose of nystatin when taken together. Others, however, have what seems to be a toxic reaction to the drug – something which is difficult to identify because of the possibility of confusion with 'die-off' symptoms.

Nizoral/ketoconazole

Nizoral is not as safe to use as nystatin and amphotericin, because it can cause liver damage. This is linked to the fact that it has been shown to be well absorbed from the gut into the bloodstream. It should not be used, therefore, without regular monitoring of liver function. Doctors who rely solely on anti-fungal drugs may be tempted to use it because it is more effective systemically.

Diflucan/fluconazole

Diflucan is a derivative of ketoconazole. When this drug was first marketed in 1989 it was claimed that one pill would mop up all candida infestation! The manufacturers now say that it is possible to take it in smaller doses over three to six months. It would appear that they have extended the time-span because of the failure of Diflucan to have any effect on one day. Diflucan is expensive, and unnecessary when there are natural alternatives available that have been shown to be effective over time.

Enzyme potentiated desensitisation

EPD was developed by Dr Len McEwan in 1966. It was originally intended for hayfever sufferers, but its use was extended to others with food allergy. It is now being used as part of an overall treatment for ME and candidiasis by some doctors. Minute doses, along homoeopathic principles, are made from extracts of most foods, which are combined with an enzyme. When applied by scraping a patch of skin, it is supposed to activate the immune system to respond. Treatments in the beginning are every two months, but the time in between usually extends if food tolerance gets better.

Reactions at first can be very severe; some people have become suicidal and others very weak and unable to eat without severe problems. On the other hand, others claim to have been helped by this treatment. Practitioners who use EPD treatments privately put forward the argument that financial costs decrease over time. Dr Jenkins at the Royal Homoeopathic Hospital provides EPD on the National Health. Most doctors giving this treatment also recommend nystatin to be taken beforehand and/or at the same time.

MAKING CHOICES

In the real world most of us have to make choices dependent on financial resources. If you think you have candidiasis and you want to treat it, changing your diet and taking Mycopryl, allicin if necessary, and digestive enzymes (all supplied by BioCare) would be a good starting point. It would be worth finding out how open your GP is to diagnosing and treating candidiasis. Previously, many GPs were concerned about the long-term effects of nystatin; using natural products should get over that problem (all BioCare's products are available on

NHS prescription, using an ACB5 form for borderline substances).

It is not advisable to treat yourself with nutritional supplements because of the dangers of causing further imbalances. However, some doctors do not recognise the value of supplementation, and if you are unable to afford the supplements plus a consultation with a nutritionally aware doctor or practitioner, you may be tempted to go it alone.

If you need the treatment to be simplified for you, some practitioners are providing a postal service for candida sufferers. Jo Hampton has put together a Candida Control Pack, which contains one month's supply of a vitamin and mineral supplement in capsule form (more expensive, but more effective), odourless garlic tablets, Mycopryl and probiotics, together with a set of instructions (for example, probiotics should not be taken at the same time as garlic), a diet sheet and a symptom record sheet. She also recommends a regular lymphatic massage as part of the recuperative treatment. Buying Mycopryl this way is slightly more expensive than buying from the manufacturer direct.

Having candidiasis is not easy. As with any condition that is 'new', it takes time for appropriate and safe treatment to evolve. The case studies reflect the fact that late diagnosis and piecemeal treatment make recovery difficult. In such a situation there is eventual recognition of other forms of self-help – dealing with emotional issues which may help to activate our own healing process.

20 LETTING GO OF ANGER AND FEAR, AND TAKING CONTROL

Orthodox medicine and unenlightened alternative medicine prolong illness by labelling the patient as ill rather than in need. But an important part of getting better is to be made, by force of circumstance or by appropriate help, to assume responsibility for your own health rather than relying solely on outside interventions.

There is no doubt that there is a connection between the mind and the body, whereby one's thoughts and emotions can effect biochemical changes. An obvious example is the brain's ability to trigger adrenaline release from the adrenal glands. This hormone release results in blood sugar levels being raised, as stores are released from the liver, i.e. energy reserves are mobilised so that they are available for the muscles; the eyes are prepared for night vision as the pupils are dilated; heart rate and blood pressure increase, allowing oxygen and nutrients to be circulated to the muscles and brain more rapidly; and the blood supply to the gut is much reduced, increasing the supply to the limbs and brain. This is called the fight and flight response, and would originally have been used to cope with physical danger; this mobilisation of the body's reserves would have been utilised by staying to cope with the danger or running away, after which the body would have returned to its normal state. For example, the blood supply to the gut would have been increased to its usual level to facilitate digestion.

Nowadays, though, this response is triggered far more by stress and emotional imbalance than it is by danger. And in most situations we are not able to resolve the stress – we are not able to fight or run away – so the reserves we have drawn on are not utilised, and the body remains in an almost constant state of preparedness for 'danger'.

The point is, though, that if normal biochemical processes are disrupted by emotional states, they can also be retuned to optimum efficiency once the 'on guard' response is allowed to rest. Dorothy Rowe, in her book *Beyond Fear*, examines the processes by which we handle fear. What she has to say has direct relevance to our concern with how the mind affects the body. If we lie to ourselves and if we lack self-confidence, our world of meaning is not consistent and we feel we are unable to meet danger with courage and mastery. 'Then we have to choose a defense against fear.' We may not be able to eradicate fear, but we can learn to deal with fear so that we are no longer overwhelmed by it. At the root of everything, dictating our response to the world, is how strongly we feel we have a right to exist.

Dr John Harrison repeats this theme in his book *Love Your Disease. It's Keeping You Healthy*:

> Acting upon the messages given to us in childhood we see ourselves as someone with an unqualified right to exist, a qualified right to exist or no right to exist. Mental attitude affects our body chemistry.

He goes on to suggest that by becoming ill we spare ourselves the trauma of examining those aspects of ourselves we have chosen to suppress. The doctor/patient relationship becomes one of earnestly searching for cure, while the patient's intention to maintain the disease is ignored by mutual agreement. Thus, the patient/doctor relationship is founded on a mutually sustaining fear: the patient fears taking responsibility for who she is, and the doctor fears not having the answers. Doctors need the illusion of possessing greater knowledge and understanding than the patient. Technology provides that mystique. The doctor can hide behind technical terminology, and the patient can gratefully hand over responsibility for her own recovery.

However, Dr Harrison argues that it is those doctors who do not play the game who help their patients most. But having taken the decision to get well, some people may experience fear when encouraged to start to take responsibility for themselves;

during this transition stage they may need temporarily to rely on the authority, status and protection of the doctor.

Psychotherapy is an alternative but it does not get us nearer to health if the therapist is allowed to assume responsibility. If in psychotherapy we seek the unconditional love of perfect parents, we deny ourselves the opportunity of discovering the parent within ourselves. By being afraid to be responsible we set up an endless search for someone or something to take care of us.

Philippa Pullar, a well-known writer on healing, agrees that wanting to be healed should include the willingness to change. She notes the significance of the fact that medicine-men ask their patients why they want to be well before they begin to heal them. The answer demonstrates whether or not they want to go back to the same pattern of behaviour that led to the illness in the first place. Philippa Pullar's own practice as a healer has shown that there are always some people who are unwilling to change because they need their illness, even though they may not be consciously aware of the fact.

I interviewed Lily Cornford, a healer, who at 83 still works six days a week. Whilst waiting I was fascinated to observe two healers working on a dog who had come into the waiting room supported only by two front legs and two wheels at the back. A train had paralysed its back legs, and the distraught owner had refused to have it put down. Instead, for the previous three months the dog had come once a week to Lily's clinic. After ten minutes, during which the healers worked together laying their hands on the dog, the dog got up and walked on four legs. It was not an instant cure, and the dog clearly needed to practise its regained skill, but it was a vivid testimony to the sometimes uncomfortable truth that all things cannot necessarily be explained. This story shows, for those not too sceptical to believe it, that there are techniques which heal and regenerate beyond the psychology of health.

Moving from animals to people, we come back to underlying emotional blocks. To use Lily's own words:

> It is fear that holds people back. Fear of the unknown. If you can only overcome an infinitesimal amount of fear you are doing the world a service. When you treat children there is no fear, unless the adult has instilled fear into them.
>
> A lot of our healing is talking. There isn't anyone that

walks through that door and stays that doesn't change. But we never ask them to change, it just happens. One of the energies that we give here is the unconditional energy of love. The other energy that we use when we heal is colour. And we always give hope. Everywhere else they are not given hope.

Lily also uses hypnosis.

With hypnosis I relax the person into a nice calm state. I act like a farmer sowing seed. You can stand and watch but you can't do anything about it. I put two seed thoughts into their subconscious mind to look at and nourish and ultimately to present to the conscious mind. First is the elimination of fear. Fear stops everyone from attaining full potential – physical, emotional and mental fear. It's nonsense that we all have to have fear to get our adrenaline glands working. Adrenals work with joy, laughter, music and love. The second seed thought is the growing of inner strength and inner confidence. With these we can become our true selves. That beautiful self, higher self, call it what you like.

One woman in hypnosis had a fear and didn't know what it was. She was 40. We came down the years in tens, and went into the womb, and it was not her fear, it was her mother's. She didn't want her. We sat and talked about it, and she knew immediately that it was the truth. It's just releasing what we already know from the unconscious.

Louise Hay, a healer and writer who overcame her own terminal cancer, also talks about healing as a willingness to change inside.

I can almost tell when people first come to me if they're going to make it or not. I look at their attitude towards themselves and their willingness to commit themselves to whatever they must do to heal themselves. We have to be willing to fight our fear, which dissolves when we allow the love that is within all of us to surface.

If healing is about change, one way to initiate such change is to accept yourself. Having done that, your relationship to others is changed too. If we don't accept ourselves we live in fear of other people. Unacknowledged fear is usually followed by anger.

Dorothy Rowe, a practising psychologist, finds that many of her patients, in looking for a new self, do not realise that that part of themselves which they despise is in fact the source of their creativity, freedom and individuality. Sometimes we go through a great deal of pain and suffering before we realise that we must care for ourselves.

So, if we need to be alert to our own role in creating illness, there is a parallel demand for change on the part of those trained to help us. Bernie Siegal MD, in his book *Love, Medicine and Miracles*, describes how his adoption of the doctors' standard professional defence against pain and failure led to unhappiness, and how his aspirations changed from being a cancer physician to wanting a job that involved people.

> I considered becoming a teacher – or a veterinarian, because veterinarians can hug their patients . . . Then it finally dawned on me. All this time I had been dealing in cases, charts, diseases, remedies, staff, and prognoses, instead of people. I'd thought of my patients merely as machines I had to repair . . . Too often the pressure squeezes out our native compassion.
>
> I tried to 'step out from behind my desk' and open the door to my heart as well as my office. Now I literally have my desk against the wall so my patients and I are in position to face each other as equals . . . I began encouraging my patients to call me by my first name. In the beginning it was quite scary to be just Bernie, not Dr Siegal – to meet others as a person, not a label. It meant I had to like myself and deserve respect for what I did rather than what I'd learned at school. But the change was well worth it. It's a simple yet effective way to break down the barrier between doctor and patient . . . I no longer shielded myself emotionally from the scenes of sadness I had to witness each day . . . First I began hugging patients, figuring they need my reassurance. Later I found I was saying 'I need to hug you,' so that I could go on.

Dr Siegal (it's difficult to say 'Bernie'!) distinguishes between detached concern, his former mode, and rational concern, which allows the expression of feeling without impairing ability to make decisions. He divides cancer patients into three groups. The 15–20 per cent who want to die; the 60–70 per cent in the middle who act the way the doctor wants them to act because it's easier to have the work done for them; and the 15–

20 per cent who are exceptional because they refuse to play the victim, and educate themselves to become specialists in their own care. He suggests that the patients who are labelled difficult or uncooperative are those most likely to get well.

Recognising his role as a teacher, he was still nevertheless amazed by the results when people who had been stable or deteriorating for a long time suddenly began to get well. He didn't understand why, and had to allow them to explain.

> 'We're getting better,' they told me, 'because you've given us hope and put us in control of our lives. You don't understand because you're a doctor. Sit and be patient.' I did and they became my teachers.

The majority of doctors will shy away from this different approach, and there is nothing in their training to encourage them to do otherwise. I suspect that one factor in the minds of British doctors would be the patients' horror if doctors dropped their titles and pushed back their desks. Clearly, not only doctors need re-educating.

An illustration of how a medical journalist shifted his view of health and healing is provided by Neville Hodgkinson. He writes in his book *Will To Be Well* of how in 1980 he was asked to write an article about multiple sclerosis. At the time he didn't know much about it, but like any experienced journalist he was able to present the 'facts' as if he did. The article was headlined 'A crippling disease that has no cure'. A few days later a response arrived from British playwright Roger MacDougall, then a professor in the University of California's theatre department. At the time of writing he was 70, in good health and with no signs of disability. At 45 he had been a wheelchair-bound victim of MS with only a short time to live. Neville Hodgkinson realised that his original regurgitation of 'medical mythology' bore no relation to the 'vital, health-promoting, self-reliant way of thinking' embodied in the letter. The letter is a good illustration of the attitude needed by sufferers of many other illnesses. First the courage, determination and optimism to go against conventional thinking; second the intuitive sense that getting to the cause may be more to do with digestion and nutrition than looking at the end result symptoms; and, third, the viewing of illness as a process that needs, not a cure but, more realistically, on-going control.

> How come at the age of seventy I am living a healthy, happy, symptom-free existence in sunny California? Simply because I refused to believe in the medical myth . . . I reasoned out the condition afresh, starting from scratch, realised that I was not, as doctors tend to postulate, a sort of living cadaver, but was more usefully to be regarded as a biochemical process . . . I set about discovering and correcting the various food allergies and chemical deficiencies which were preventing my metabolism from functioning properly. Over the next ten years or so my symptoms gradually melted away, like snow in the summer, until now I am normal again. Of course I am not 'cured' – simply restored to normalcy. Were I to revert to my old eating habits, I would once again suffer from the so-called disease of multiple sclerosis . . .
>
> Neurologists are wasting their time researching the condition. It should be left to the biochemists. Neurologists would do their patients much more service if they would forget the nervous tissue which is where the condition ends and concentrate on the metabolism – on nutrition and chemical make-up. That way they might learn to help people instead of simply diagnosing them and then shrugging helplessly as they watch them degenerate.

Neville Hodgkinson concludes that Roger MacDougall, and many others who have learnt how to control MS, succeed not primarily because they have the ability to stick rigidly to dietary change, but because of a mental attitude committed to banishing the illness from their lives.

It is interesting that sufferers of a 'legitimate' illness, cancer, are moving towards a recognition of their emotional links to their illness and their ability to get well. Cancer self-help groups were set up because of sufferers' needs to add to or reject conventional treatment, and to provide, through counselling, healing, visualisation and nutritional changes, a new way of fighting the disease and a new way of relating to others. These aids to healing are not used in isolation from other therapies, but they are seen by many as essential tools in the fight to get well. Raymond Hitchcock's book *Fighting Cancer* gives a vivid account of how visualisation, diet, personal change and healing contributed to his return to health.

To be sure, as with cancer, many problems of candidiasis and ME stem from inherited weaknesses and environmental overload; emotional factors may not always 'cause' the problems, but getting over them may need a recharged emotional response. The reality, of course, is that there are many external causes for both candidiasis and ME; many of the mental symptoms are organically produced or, if not, could be a result of being ill as much as the cause of it. But the external causes are cofactors, working together with varying degrees of input and depending for effect on how we respond to them at a deeper level, sometimes beyond our conscious grasp. Sufferers of candidiasis and ME are diverted from looking inward for reasons that do not apply to other 'validated' illnesses. Because of their initial need to gain recognition from scientific medicine in a desperate search for treatment, and the rejection or inappropriate treatment that ensues, their status as 'victims' is emphasised.

The modern world's ever greater dependency on medicine and the instant cure can lead to ever greater anger towards it if it fails. Left with the label of 'psychosomatic' – implying that there are more deserving illnesses which do not involve the mind – it is hardly surprising if sufferers of candidiasis give more attention to the symptoms than any underlying need for change.

As yet, in Britain, candidiasis has no public face from the point of view of the sufferers. But the self-help journals from the ME groups reveal, from different perspectives, an understandably defensive reaction to any suggestion that implicates psychological causes. When doctors deny the reality of the biochemical processes at work it is hardly an inducement to consider psychological factors. And when the debate is couched in terms of 'accusation' and smug professional distance, there is even less chance of calling a truce.

Perhaps the most hopeful lesson I have learnt from interviewing sufferers of candidiasis and ME is that making the shift to recognising personal responsibility for recovery need not lead to blame, self-recrimination and guilt. On the contrary, opening up and letting go can lead to acceptance, engagement and the possibility of change.

SUMMARY

- There is a connection between the mind and the body, leading to biochemical changes.

- Accept illness. Trying to deny it will not make it go away.
- Getting better is not simply a matter of being the 'good patient' and doing what we are told. Getting better is hard work, involving the assessment of treatments and requiring internal shifts of meaning and a more realistic acceptance of self.
- Trusting our own intuitive sense of what helps may require us to assert our needs, despite 'experts' who get in the way.
- Working in partnership with doctors, therapists and practitioners requires an awareness on the part of professionals that they also have needs. Our expectations as 'patients' should not encourage those helping us to act with divine authority – our need for the perfect parent obstructs our recognition of our own potential and power within.
- Responding to the challenge of emotional change can only come about, when ill, if there is a fundamental belief in the value of health in the way we live our lives.
- Reaching for health does not mean finding a 'cure'. The healing process begins as soon as we start to think about change. Once the goal becomes looking behind fear to a new acceptance of self, the right healing environment is created.
- Shifting responsibility for the disease away from external causes, so that it also includes personal responsibility, does not imply blame or guilt. But accepting the emotional needs that are met by illness allows us to move beyond those needs, or to satisfy them in other ways.

INFORMATION, SUPPORT AND ADVICE

Action Against Allergy
Greyhound House
23–4 George Street
Richmond
Surrey TW9 1JY
A membership organisation, with a newsletter giving advice and research information. Some local groups, but not formally affiliated. Send a large SAE.

ME Action
PO Box 1302
Wells BA2 2WE
Membership organisation, with over 100 local groups, £12.50 a year, which includes three copies of their journal *Interaction* and access to the Therapy and Information Helpline. Therapy factsheets are also available on request. It also functions to sponsor research and is interested in a wide range of therapies and treatments. Candida sufferers are encouraged to join.

Foodcare Self-Help Group
181 Lymington Rd
Torquay
Devon TQ1 4BA
0803 312580
Local groups for candida sufferers, support and information.

ME Association
PO Box 8
Stanford-le-Hope
Essex SS17 8EX
A membership organisation, costing £12 a year, which includes ME Association Newsletter four times a year, and access to a 'Listening Ear' telephone advice service. There are local groups throughout the country. It is interested in the orthodox, scientific approach to ME, and is not officially behind the 'candida connection', although many members acknowledge it in their treatment.

Springhill Centre
Cuddington Road
Dinton
Aylesbury
Buckinghamshire HP18 0AD
0296 748278
Set up by Dr Nadya Coates and her husband, Hugh, Springhill provides respite and relief care for chronically sick children and young people, including those with disabling and life limiting disease. Conductive education for motor disabled people is offered. At the same time it runs seminars on diet, and candidiasis.

Hyperactive Children's Support Group
Sally Bunday
71 Whyke Lane
Chichester
West Sussex PO21 2DE
Wide experience in the treatment of candida in children. Membership includes their journal; there are many local support groups. Also supplies nutritional supplements especially formulated for children. Send an SAE.

National Society for Research into Allergy
PO Box 45
Hinckley
Leicestershire LE10 1JY
Local groups.

Women's Health and Information Centre
52 Featherstone Street
London EC1
071–251 6580
Advice and library.

Green Farm Foodwatch
Burwash Common
East Sussex TN19 7LX
0435 882482
Mail order suppliers of specialized foods.

ANTI-FUNGAL AIDS AND NUTRITIONAL SUPPLEMENTS

BioCare
17 Pershore Road South
Birmingham B30 3EE
021–433 3727

Suppliers of Mycopryl, Digest Aid (digestive enzymes), Colon Care, Oxy-Pro, Bio-Acidophilus, Artemisia Complex, Butyric Acid Complex, Enteroplex, GLA Complex, Cervagyn, Cervagyn Plus, Cystoplex, vitamins and minerals. (All BioCare's products are now available on prescription using an ACBS form.)

Blackmores
Unit 7, Poyle Tech Centre
Willow Road
Poyle, Colnbrook
Bucks SL3 0PD
0753 683815
Suppliers of Garlix

Lamberts Healthcare Ltd
1 Lamberts Road
Tunbridge Wells
Kent TN2 3EQ
0892 513116
Suppliers of Super Acidophilus Plus

Advanced Nutrition Ltd
8 Chilston Road
Tunbridge Wells
Kent TN4 9LT
0892 515927
Suppliers of nutritional supplements, digestive enzymes, and amino-acids. A good source of linseed oil and *aloe vera* juice.

Gerrard House
3 Wickham Road
Boscombe
Bournemouth
Dorset BH7 6JX
0202 434116
Good quality herbal products.

PRACTITIONERS

I have not made a comprehensive survey of practitioners, and this list is by no means exclusive. I have only included those doctors with a more cautious approach to nystatin. Where capricin is not used by practitioners because of cost, Allicin Complex is often recommended as a good alternative.

Leon Chaitow (naturopath and osteopath)
The Hale Clinic
7 Park Crescent
London W1
071–631 0156

Dr Gwynn Davies
Nirvana
4 Calway Road
Taunton
Somerset TA1 3EQ
0823 335610

Drs. Dowson, Kenyon, Lewith
Centre for the Study of Complementary Medicine
51 Bedford Place
Southampton SO1 2DG
0703 334752

Dr Robert Erdmann
Medabolics Ltd
8 Chilston Road
Tunbridge Wells
Kent TN4 9LT
0892 542609

Dr Keith Eaton
Cadley Mews
Cadley
Marlborough
Wiltshire SN8 4NE
0672 55266

Jo Hampton (ex-sufferer who describes herself as a Natural Practitioner)
Earthdust Products
46 Wainfleet Road
Skegness
Lincolnshire PE25 3QT
0754 68336

Dr Alan Hibberd
Bayswater Clinic
25B Clanricarde Gardens
London W2 4JL
071–229 9078

Kay Hitchen (naturopath)
Natural Way (Anglesey) Ltd
Arfryn
Caergeillog
Anglesey
Gwynedd LL65 3NL
0407 741297

Dr Patrick Kingsley
72 Main Street
Osgathorpe
Leicestershire LE12 9TA
0530 223622

Maggie la Tourelle (kinesiologist and counsellor)
58 Leverton Street
London NW5 2NU
071–485 4215

Linda Lazarides (nutritional counsellor)
Neals Yard Therapy Rooms
No 2 Neals Yard
Covent Garden
London WC2
071–379 7662

Dr John Mansfield
Burghwood Clinic
34 Brighton Road
Banstead
Surrey SM7 1BS
07373 61177

Dr Peter Maslin
30A Church Street
Stornoway
Isle of Lewis
Scotland PA87 2JD
0851 2010

Erica White (ex-sufferer and nutritional counsellor)
22 Leigh Hall Road
Leigh-on-Sea
Essex SS9 1RN
0702 72085

OTHER PRACTITIONERS

British College of Naturopathy and Osteopathy
6 Netherhall Gardens
London NW3
071–435 7830
Reduced fees for supervised student consultations and free treatment for children.

Confederation of Healing Organizations
113 Hampstead Way
London NW11 7JN

Colonics International Association
26 Sea Road
Boscombe
Bournemouth
Dorset BH5 1DF

Kinesiology Federation
Touch for Health Centre
30 Sudley Road
Bognor Regis
West Sussex PO21 1ER
0243 583350 (Daphne Clarke)

The Shiatsu Society
19 Langside Park
Kilbarchan
Renfrewshire
Scotland PA10 2EP
05057 4657
List of qualified shiatsu therapists.

Acupuncture
There are many different schools of acupuncture, but a listing of practitioners can be obtained from:

The Institute for Complementary Medicine
21 Portland Place
London W1N 3AF

TESTS AND SCREENING

Biolab
The Stone House
9 Weymouth Street
London W1N 3FF
071–636 5959/5905
For assessment of nutritional status, a doctor's referral is needed.

Bio-Screen Ltd
Broadway House
14 Mount Pleasant Road
Tunbridge Wells
Kent TN1 1QU
0892 542012
Urine tests for status of digestive enzymes and presence of systemic candidiasis. Practitioner's referral necessary.

BIBLIOGRAPHY

The Allergy Connection, B. Paterson, Thorsons, Wellingborough, 1985.

The Amino Revolution, R. Erdmann and M. Jones, Century, London, 1987.

Antifungal Chemotherapy, D.C.E. Speller (ed.), John Wiley, Chichester, 1980.

Beyond Fear, D. Rowe, Fontana, London, 1987.

The Biogenic Diet, L. Kenton, Arrow, London, 1986.

The Bitter Pill, E. Grant, Corgi, London, 1985.

Candida: The Symptoms, The Causes, The Cure, Luc de Schepper, 1986. Available from: 2901 Wilshire Boulevard, Suite 435, Santa Monica, CA 90403, USA. Revised British edition, *Candida: Diet Against It,* Foulsham, Slough, 1989.

Candida Albicans: Could Yeast Be Your Problem? Leon Chaitow, Thorsons, Wellingborough, 1985.

Candida and Candidosis, F.C. Odds, Baillière Tindall, London, 1988.

Candida and Thrush, Dr. George T. Lewith, BioMed Publications Ltd., 52 Northfield Road, Birmingham B30 1JH or from BioCare, 1990.

Chronic Fatigue and the Yeast Syndrome, W.G. Crook, Professional Books, 1992.

Clinical Microbiology, E.J. Stokes and G.L. Ridgway (eds), Edward Arnold, London, 1987.

The Complete Guide to Food Allergy and Intolerance, J. Brostoff and L. Gamlin, Bloomsbury, London, 1989.

Conquering Cystitis, P. Kingsley, Abaco Publishing, 72 Main Street, Osgathorpe, Leicestershire, LE12 9TA, 1987.

Cured to Death, A. Melville and C. Johnson, Secker & Warburg, London, 1982.

Everywoman: A Gynaecological Guide For Life, D. Llewellyn-Jones, Faber & Faber, London, 1985.

Fighting Cancer, Raymond Hitchcock, Angel Press, 1989. Available from: PO Box 60, East Wittering, West Sussex, PO20 8RA.

The Food Factor, B. Griggs, Penguin, London, 1986.
Gentle Giants, P. Brohn, Century, London, 1987.
Living With ME, C. Shepherd, Cedar, London, 1989.
Love, Medicine and Miracles, B. Siegal, Arrow, London, 1988.
Love Your Disease, J. Harrison, Angus & Robertson, London, 1986.
Maximum Immunity, M.A. Weiner, Gateway Books, Bath, 1986.
ME: How To Live With It, A. Macintyre, Unwin Hyman, London, 1989.
The Missing Diagnosis, C. Orion Truss, 1982. Available from: PO Box 26508, Birmingham, AL 35226, USA.
Multiple Sclerosis, J. Graham, Thorsons, Wellingborough, 1987.
Not All In The Mind, R. Mackarness, Pan, London, 1976.
Nutritional Medicine, S. Davies and A. Stewart, Pan, London, 1987.
Overcoming Addictions, J. Pleshette, Thorsons, Wellingborough, 1989.
The Psychological Consequences of Cerebral Disorder, W.A. Lishman, Blackwell, Oxford, 1987.
Spiritual and Lay Healing, P. Pullar, Penguin, London, 1988.
Stone Age Diet, Leon Chaitow, Macdonald Optima, London, 1987.
Thorsons Introductory Guide to Kinesiology, Maggie la Tourelle with Anthea Courtenay, Thorsons, 1992
Tissue Cleansing Through Bowel Management, Bernard Jensen, (1981), Available from: Box 52, Route 1, Escondido, CA 92025, USA.
Will To Be Well, N. Hodgkinson, Hutchinson, London, 1984.
Women and The Crisis in Sex Hormones, B. Seaman and G. Seaman, Bantam, New York, 1981.
A World Without AIDS, Leon Chaitow and Simon Martin, Thorsons, Wellingborough, 1989.
The Wound and the Doctor: Healing, Technology and Power in Modern Medicine, Glin Bennet, Secker & Warburg, London, 1987.
The Yeast Connection, W.G. Crook, Vintage, London, 1986.
The Yeast Syndrome, J.P. Trowbridge and M. Walker, Bantam, New York, 1987.
You Can Heal Your Life, L. Hay, Eden Grove Editions, London, 1988.

INDEX

Action Against Allergy, ix
addiction, 94–103
AIDS: 54, 77, 145
allergies, 40–5
aloe vera juice, 159
alternative medicine, 168
amphotericin B, 164–5
antibiotics, 94–103
Apich syndrome, 31–2
Association of Carers, 75
Association for Improvement in Maternity Services, 60

Beard, 71
bifidobacteria, 7
bio-kinesiology, 44;
Biocare, 166
biotin, 159
birth control pill, 30–1, 85
The Bitter Pill, 30
bowels, elimination process, 11–14
Brostoff, Dr Jonathan, 21, 44, 147
Bunday, Sally, 57
butyric acid, 161

candida albicans: advice group, 55; better habits, 155; diagnosis and help, 143–4; killing off, 156–7; ME connection, 76–8; men, 29–30, 32–3, 135–42; opportunistic invader, 1–6; picking up clues, 27–9; questionnaire, 35–9; symptoms, 26–7, 33–5; tests for, 144–5; what it does, 24–39
candidiasis: difficult to test, 4; doctors deny, 3
capricin, 156–7
carbohydrates, 151
cells, 16–18
Chaitow, Leon, ix, 53, 77
childbirth, choices in, 59–60
Clinical Ecology Group, 43
Coates, Dr Nadya, 2, 13
colon, 11
colonics, 159–60
Colquohoun, Irene, 57
Cornford, Lily, 170–71
cortisone, 62
Crook, Dr William, 53
cystitis, 25–6

Davis, Adelle, 124
de Schepper, Luc, 46–7, 155
DES, 61
diagnoses, mistaken, 145–6
diagnosis, 143–4
dietary advice, 148–56
digestion, 8–11, 69
digestive enzymes, 153–4
Downing, Dr Damien, 147
drug companies, 41

enemas, 159–60
enzyme potentiated desensitisation, 165–6
Erdmann, R, 17
essential fatty acids, 152–3

fear, 170, 171
Finlay, Sue, 73

food intolerance, 34, 40–5, 69
food rotation, 154
foods: to avoid, 148–51; to eat, 151–2
Francis, Clare, 73

Galland, Dr Leo, 145
garlic, 158
gluten, 149–51
gold injections, 62
Graham, Judy, 58
Grant, Ellen, 30
Green Farm Nutrition Centre, 54
Griggs, Barbara, 63

Harrison, Dr John, 169
Hay, Louise, 171
healers, 128–30
healing, 170
Hitchcock, Raymond, 174
Hodgkinson, Neville, 173, 174
Hood, Jimmy MP, 73
hormone function, 29–30
hyperactivity, 57–8
hyperventilation, 74
hynosis, 171
hypoglycaemia, 63–6

immune system: 1, 31; how it works, 16–18
immunotherapy, 52
interleukin–1 beta, 70
Issels, Dr Josef, 3, 52

Jensen, Bernard, 8
Johnson, Colin, 57
Jones, M, 17

ketoconazole, 165
Kingsley, Dr Patrick, 25, 43

lactobacillus acidophilus, 7
Lane, Sir Arbuthnot, 11–12
Lehmann, Stephanie, ix

McCarrison Society, 43
McEvedy, 71
Macintyre, Ann, 68
Mackarness, Dr Richard, 42
Mansfield, Dr John, 43
Martin, Simon, 77
massage, 130–4
ME: 48, 55; AIDS, 77; candida connection, 76–8; mass hysteria, 71, 72; media, ME, 67–78; symptoms, 68–72
ME Action Campaign, 73
ME Association, 73, 76
Melville, Arabella, 57
milk, 151
minerals, 161–2
Monro, Dr Jean, 43, 91
mould, 156
mould-containing foods, 151
multiple sclerosis, 43, 58–9
myalgic encephalomyelitis, *see* ME
Mycopryl, 156–7

Natural Childbirth Trust, 60
New Health Society, 12
nizoral, 165
nystatin, 163–4

Odds, F.C., 49–50
oleic acid, 159
Oliver, Judith, 75
organic vegetables, 154
oxy–pro, 158–9

Paterson, Barbara, 41, 42
Pfeiffer, Dr Carl, 161
postnatal depression, 85
probiotic supplementation, 160
psychological factors, 5, 26
Pullar, Philippa, 170
pyroluria, 161

Ramsay, Dr, 72

Randolph, Dr Theron, 41
Richmond, Caroline, 65
rotation of food, 154
Rowe, Dorothy, 172

Saifer, Dr Phyllis, 31
Shepherd, Dr Charles, 16, 56, 76
Siegal, Bernie, 172
Smith, Dr Tony, 75
Speller, 48
Springhill Cancer Centre, 2, 149–51
steroids, 31
stilboestrol, 61
Stoppard, Dr Miriam, 75
supplements, 162–3

terminology, 68
tests for candidiasis, 144–5
thalidomide, 61
thrush, 24–5
Tissue Cleansing through Bowel Management, 8
toxins, 2
tranquillisers, 94–103
Trowbridge, 31, 35
Truss, Dr C. Orian, 27

Valium, 62
vitamins, 161–2
von Pirquet, Clemens, 40

Walker, 31, 35
Weiner, M.A., 54
Weiner, Michael, 15
Wessely, Simon, 78
Winger, Dr Edward, 32

yeast, 151

UNDERSTANDING ENDOMETRIOSIS
Caroline Hawkridge

Written in conjunction with the Endometriosis Society, this book provides the most up-to-date and comprehensive information on the causes, diagnosis and treatment of this increasingly common gynaecological disorder.
'Essential reading for sufferers and GPs, as well as doctors and nurses working in the gynaecological field.' **Nursing Times**

0-356-15447-5

THE MENOPAUSE
Coping With The Change
Dr Jean Coope

This invaluable guide answers frequently asked questions and provides practical advice on how to make the menopause a change for the better.

0-356-14511-1

DIABETES AND PREGNANCY
Anna Knopfler

Diabetic mother Anna Knopfler provides clear information and reassurance on all aspects of diabetic management, pregnancy and childbirth.

0-356-15189-1

AVOIDING OSTEOPOROSIS
Dr Allan Dixon and Dr Anthony Woolf

Osteoporosis causes pain and disability in one in four post-menopausal women; this practical guide examines causes and symptoms and outlines methods of prevention and treatment.

0-356-15445-9

THE BREAST BOOK
John Cochrane MS, FRCS and Dr Anne Szarewski

Comprehensive information and advice on all aspects of breast health and care, including breastfeeding and breast cancer.

0-356-15416-5

SELF-HELP WITH PMS
Escape from the Prison of Premenstrual Tension
Dr Michelle Harrison

A positive approach provides clear, up-to-date advice on the problems of, and cures for, premenstrual syndrome.
'. . . a thought-provoking and valuable book on a little understood subject.' **Health Visitor**
'. . . a lifeline for anyone trying to pull themselves out of the misery of premenstrual tension.' **Guardian**

0-356-12559-9

CYSTITIS
A Woman Doctor's Guide to Prevention and Treatment
Dr Kathryn Schrotenboer with Sue Berkman

50% of women can expect to experience cystitis at some time; designed to help women formulate their own prevention plan, this book explains how to treat, and perhaps even more importantly how to avoid, recurrent attacks.

0-356-15448-3

MENOPAUSE THE NATURAL WAY
Dr Sadya Greenwood

Correcting myths and explaining all medical details, this comprehensive book answers all the questions that are asked about the menopause.

0-356-12561-0

MISCARRIAGE
Margaret Leroy

'clear, sensible information. . . . I would not hesitate to recommend it to anyone who wants to know more about miscarriage.' **Nursing Times**
'Anyone who has experienced a miscarriage should be directed to (this) book.' **The Lancet**

0-356-12888-1

ALTERNATIVE MATERNITY
Nicky Wesson

From acupuncture to cranial osteopathy to medical herbalism, this book provides a comprehensive guide to the range of alternative remedies and therapies available for both mother and baby at all stages of maternity. Covers conception, pregnancy, childbirth and early infant care.

0-356-15412-2

ENCYCLOPAEDIA OF NATURAL MEDICINE
Michael Murray N.D. and Joseph Pizzorno N.D.

Based on the work and research done at the John Bastyr College of Naturopathic Medicine in America, the *Encyclopaedia of Natural Medicine* is a fully comprehensive guide and reference to all aspects of natural treatment for illness. It explains the principles of natural medicine and their application, in addition to defining a preventative, healthy lifestyle.
The coverage of specific health problems – ranging from acne to candidiasis, depression to gallstones, irritable bowel syndrome to osteoporosis, sinus infection to varicose veins – is extensive, and details the relevant naturopathic treatments, ensuring full usefulness both in the home or by practitioners.

0-356-17218-X

ALTERNATIVE HEALTH GUIDES

MEDITATION

Erica Smith and Nicholas Wilks

Meditation is a state of inner stillness which has been cultivated by mystics for thousands of years. The main reason for its recent popularity is that regular practice has been found to improve mental and physical health, largely due to its role in alleviating stress.

0-356-209954

HYPNOSIS

Ursula Markham

Hypnosis has a remarkable record of curing a wide range of ills. Ursula Markham, a practising hypnotherapist, explains how, by releasing inner tensions, hypnosis can help people to heal themselves.

0-356-209962

CHIROPRACTIC

Susan Moore

This guide to chiropractic concentrates on the actual treatment itself, seen from a patients point of view. In a straightforward way, it answers all your questions about chiropractic, as well as providing background information about this popular therapy. The author is a practising chiropractor, well aware of the concerns of first-time patients.

0–356–124339

HERBAL MEDICINE
Anne McIntyre
Herbal medicine has been known for thousands of years. It is an entirely natural system of medicine which relies on the therapeutic quality of plants to enhance the body's recuperative powers, and so bring health – without any undesirable side effects.

0–356–124290

All Optima books are available at your bookshop or newsagent, or can be ordered from the following address:
Little, Brown and Company (UK) Limited,
P.O. Box 11,
Falmouth,
Cornwall TR10 9EN.

Alternatively you may fax your order to the above address.
Fax No. 0326 376423.

Payments can be made as follows: cheque, postal order (payable to Little, Brown and Company) or by credit cards, Visa/Access. Do not send cash or currency. UK customers and B.F.P.O. please allow £1.00 for postage and packing for the first book, plus 50p for the second book, plus 30p for each additional book up to a maximum charge of £3.00 (7 books plus).

Overseas customers including Ireland, please allow £2.00 for the first book plus £1.00 for the second book, plus 50p for each additional book.

NAME (Block Letters) ....

....

ADDRESS ....

....

....

☐ I enclose my remittance for ________

☐ I wish to pay by Access/Visa Card

Number

Card Expiry Date